ADVANCE PRAISE

"This thoughtful, engaging, comprehensive guide brings to life how insights and techniques from somatic psychotherapies can deepen and enrich psychedelic-assisted treatment. The authors' extensive experience with all of these modalities shines through on every page with evocative case examples, easy-to-access experiential exercises, and clear, step-by-step, practical guidance. Humble, honest, and sensible, this book is essential reading for clinicians wishing to work with psychedelics or guide clients."

—**Ronald D. Siegel, PsyD,** author of *The Extraordinary Gift of Being Ordinary: Finding Happiness Right Where You Are*, assistant professor of psychology (part-time), Harvard Medical School

"As interest in psychedelics continues to grow, so do the questions surrounding their effectiveness, potential, and risks. Mischke-Reeds and Sylvae make a compelling case for the profound promise these medicines hold—while emphasizing that true transformation hinges on thoughtful preparation, skilled guidance, and intentional integration.

In this timely and essential volume, the authors illuminate the critical role of grounding psychedelic experiences in present-moment body sensations and emotional awareness. Their somatic approach offers a powerful contribution to the evolving field of psychedelic therapy. A must-read for both those embarking on their own healing journeys and the therapists supporting them."

—**Peter A. Levine, PhD,** author of *In an Unspoken Voice* and *An Autobiography of Trauma: A Healing Journey*

"*Embodied Psychedelic Therapy* highlights the essential role of the body in psychedelic healing. Somatic therapy recognizes that transformation doesn't occur through insight alone, it must move through the body, expressing what words often cannot. This guide offers clinicians practical tools to support bottom-up processing, helping clients release trauma, integrate profound experiences, and trust their innate healing intelligence. Rooted in decades of somatic practice, *Embodied Psychedelic Therapy* is a timely and essential contribution to the evolving field of psychedelic-assisted therapy."

—**Rick Doblin, PhD,** founder and president, MAPS

"*Embodied Psychedelic Therapy* is a comprehensive and practical guide to psychedelic therapy. Grounded in Hakomi and Somatic Experiencing therapies, the authors bring a depth of experience in working with the 'indissoluble unity of body and mind.' Increasing interest in the healing potential of psychedelics has brought concerns about ethical and safe use. This book will be invaluable in preparing practitioners to use them effectively, skillfully, and wisely."

—**Annie Mithoefer, BSN and Michael Mithoefer, MD,** former therapists and trainers for MAPS clinical trials of MDMA-assisted psychotherapy for PTSD

EMBODIED PSYCHEDELIC THERAPY

EMBODIED PSYCHEDELIC THERAPY
A SOMATIC GUIDE

MANUELA MISCHKE-REEDS
JOSHUA SYLVAE

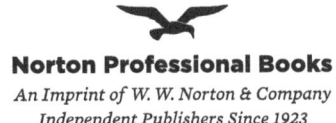

Norton Professional Books
An Imprint of W. W. Norton & Company
Independent Publishers Since 1923

This book is a general information resource for current or prospective professional providers and facilitators of psychedelic therapy, which means therapy while under the influence of psychedelic drugs. The guidelines and recommendations in this book are intended to supplement, not substitute for, appropriate training or clinical supervision. No technique or recommendation is guaranteed to be safe or effective in all circumstances. Standards of clinical practice and protocol vary in different practice settings and change over time.

The names of all patients mentioned have been changed and identifying details changed or omitted, and some patients and some session transcripts are composites. Nothing in this book constitutes or shall be deemed to constitute medical or legal advice. Psychedelic drugs other than ketamine are currently illegal in most states and at the federal level. Neither the publisher nor either author endorses or encourages any illegal practice. You alone are responsible for determining whether any drug that your patient wishes to take under your supervision to achieve a psychedelic state, and any drug that you recommend or provide to a patient for that purpose, is legal in the state whose law governs your practice. For advice about whether certain therapy is legal in a certain state, which state's laws apply to your practice, or how to prepare legally appropriate informed consent documents, or for any other legal advice or legal questions related to this kind of therapy, please consult an attorney with relevant expertise.

Any URLs displayed in this book link or refer to websites that existed as of press time. The publisher is not responsible for, and should not be deemed to endorse or recommend, any website other than its own or any content that it did not create. The authors, also, are not responsible for any third-party material.

Copyright © 2025 by Manuela Mischke-Reeds and Joshua Sylvae

All rights reserved
Printed in the United States of America
First Edition

Part opener art © Retroot Studio / Shutterstock

For information about permission to reproduce selections from this book, write to Permissions, W. W. Norton & Company, Inc., 500 Fifth Avenue, New York, NY 10110

For information about special discounts for bulk purchases, please contact W. W. Norton Special Sales at specialsales@wwnorton.com or 800-233-4830

Manufacturing by Lake Book Manufacturing
Production manager: Gwen Cullen

ISBN: 978-1-324-05355-2

W. W. Norton & Company, Inc., 500 Fifth Avenue, New York, NY 10110
www.wwnorton.com

W. W. Norton & Company Ltd., 15 Carlisle Street, London W1D 3BS

1 2 3 4 5 6 7 8 9 0

CONTENTS

ACKNOWLEDGMENTS IX

INTRODUCTION: INITIATIONS XI

PART I **OVERVIEW**

CHAPTER 1 THE FIELD OF PSYCHEDELIC THERAPY 5

CHAPTER 2 THE CENTRALITY OF ETHICS 19

CHAPTER 3 THE BODY IN PSYCHEDELIC THERAPY 42

CHAPTER 4 SOMATIC THERAPIES AND EXPANDED STATES 58

CHAPTER 5 ADVERSE EVENTS 78

PART II **PRE-JOURNEY WORK**

CHAPTER 6 PREPARING THE THERAPIST 103

CHAPTER 7 PREPARING THE CLIENT 122

CHAPTER 8 DESIGNING THE SPACE 150

PART III	**JOURNEY WORK**
CHAPTER 9	EMBODIED JOURNEYS 171
CHAPTER 10	TOUCH AND PSYCHEDELICS 196
CHAPTER 11	TRAUMA AND PSYCHEDELICS 222

PART IV	**POST-JOURNEY WORK**
CHAPTER 12	WHAT IS INTEGRATION? 245
CHAPTER 13	THERAPEUTIC TOOLS FOR INTEGRATION 260

PART V	**CONCLUSION**
CHAPTER 14	CULTURAL SET AND SETTING 283
CHAPTER 15	COMPLETION . . . AND BEYOND 293
	REFERENCES 305
	INDEX 319

ACKNOWLEDGMENTS

From Joshua:

My love and profound gratitude to my mentor, Dr. Ian Macnaughton, for his mischievous accompaniment and tireless efforts to educate me and improve my person. A deep bow to Peter Levine, PhD, Steven Hoskinson, Kathy Kain, PhD, Anthony "Twig" Wheeler, and the other somatics teachers who have touched my life. A hug to my BFF, Mahshid Fashandi Hager, for all the encouragement. Thanks to Claudia for guidance, and to Deborah Malmud at Norton for valuable feedback and support of this project. To my editor and dear friend, Peregrine Somerville . . . you have made me a better writer, and I don't think I could've made it without you; thanks so much! To my brother and proofreader, Garth Wadsworth: great gratitude for all you did, and for putting up with my stupid jokes. And to my friend, Manuela, I send huge thanks for manifesting this dream together!

None of this would be possible without the support and care of my wife, Lina, and our beautiful children, Amara and Cían. I love you all more than words can say.

I dedicate this book to the molecules, the people who protected them, and all the wild entities of land, sea, and sky.

May this work be of benefit to all beings.

From Manuela:

A special thank you to Deborah Malmud, our Norton editor, for enthusiastically saying yes to the vision of bringing somatic perspectives to psychedelic-assisted therapy. I deeply appreciate Marisa Solis for her professional and emotional support; I could not have done this without you. Thank you, Elen Turner, Peregrine Somerville, and Garth Wadsworth, for all the editing help.

Thanks to my husband, Michael Mischke-Reeds, who gave me the time and space to write late nights and weekends away from family time, and my sons, Kirian and Tristan, who always support me.

I hold dearly the many somatic and psychology lineages that have inspired my work, such as Emilie Conrad, Susan Harper, Ron Kurtz, and Peter Levine, and my colleagues at the Hakomi Institute. Also, I thank Janice Phelps for her kind support.

Thank you, Patricia James, for her wisdom; Laura Vaughan and Cheryl Kruse, for their loving listening ears; Staci Haines, for her counsel; and Raquel Bennett, for her encouragement.

I bow in deep gratitude to the ancient lineages of indigenous plant wisdom keepers who have inspired me and taught me humility through plant medicines.

Thank you, Joshua, for jumping into this project wholeheartedly and bringing grit and humor.

May this book be helpful to students and practitioners and help integrate somatic therapies with psychedelic medicines with humility, kindness, and ethical skills, benefiting others on their healing paths.

INTRODUCTION: INITIATIONS

Before you know what kindness is, you must lose things.
—NAOMI SHIHAB NYE

Altered states of consciousness, while potentially healing, can be challenging to negotiate. This book explores how to best support embodied journeys into psychedelic states. The insights offered here are gleaned from innumerable sources. We describe practices, ancient and modern, those proven to make the psychedelic experience safer and more beneficial. In addition to learning how to do this work from guides and teachers, though, we have also learned what *not* to do, sometimes from personal experience. In the following stories, we describe situations illustrating what to avoid when psychedelics are involved.

THE TEENAGER AMBLED THROUGH THE DISHEVELED LIVING room, tipped back each discarded mug, and downed its contents. Many of his friends had not finished their cups. The tea was strong, bitter, and tasted of earth. It was a potent batch, they'd said, and a full cup might've been too much for them. He wasn't worried, though. He'd eagerly accepted their invitation to take magic mushrooms that day. Drinking a full cup—and the remains of theirs—would not be a problem. He was 17 and had never taken psilocybin before, though he'd traversed the strange seas of lysergic acid diethylamide (LSD) on many occasions. He knew what he could handle. His friends' leavings shouldn't be wasted, he figured, so he drank them all down.

This young man yearned for a transformative experience. An artist and a revolutionary, he hungered for states of consciousness that could help make sense of a world he found incomprehensible. He'd puzzled for years at the cruelty and oppression adults around him accepted as normal, and had come to appreciate psychedelics for their mind-opening and expansive qualities. He looked forward to a day of connecting with his friends and breaking through the mundane reality he found so distasteful.

Waiting for the mushrooms to kick in, he perused his friend's bookshelf. One title stood out among the rest: *The Little Prince*. He began to leaf through it. He smiled. A seamless blend of childlike wonder and deep philosophical insights shone forth from its pages. As the drug took hold, the book became a magnificent trove of wisdom, and he devoured the story. With the help of this singular book he was unlocking a set of hidden truths at the very center of reality.

His friends announced they were leaving. He knit his brow, confused. They were all experienced mushroom takers, and feeling the forest calling, they headed out to the woods around The Evergreen State College where a few of them studied. Would he join them? He peered down at the book in his hands. He was *on to something*, and didn't want to leave the book or the transformative process it had initiated. Watching the group depart he was sure he'd made the right choice to be alone. Something was happening here. This was *important*.

As he pored over the pages, things began to change. The insights rushed in faster and faster, and he struggled to keep up with the blitz of thoughts flaring forth. He finished the book, and though new layers of meaning were still being revealed, the flurry of mental activity had left him dizzy. Each moment felt more significant than the moment before. He blinked, shook his head. He *had* to stay coherent enough to collect each new truth being offered, but his body felt strangely warped, and his vision was getting more and more distorted. It was all becoming a bit too intense, and he began to worry about where things were going.

Then all at once a dreadful thought entered his mind: "What if I can't make it stop?" The helplessness and overwhelm that flooded through him in that moment was but the first of what would be many panic attacks, that day and for many years beyond it.

He burst out onto the porch, panting, and tried to get his bearings. The noise and bustling of cars and people crushed in around him. People on the street would know he was high and they'd surely report him to the police. He winced, rushed back inside, but the experience had now become terrifying and he had no one to help him make sense of what was happening.

He suspected he'd gone insane, truly and irrevocably, and started to imagine what his ruined life would look like now. Raised on stories like *One Flew Over the Cuckoo's Nest*, he knew he didn't want to end up a zombified mental patient. He was an anarchist, a staunch opponent of incarceration, and would never allow himself to be caged. But his situation looked dire, indeed. He huddled in a ball as the waves of dread washed over him, desperate for something to make his suffering stop, convinced he'd crossed a threshold he'd never return from.

Sometime later, his friend Sofia came home to the crash pad.

She'd not been there that morning, and had no idea what was happening. The young man sat her down and calmly explained the situation as he saw it.

"I've lost my mind, and I can't allow myself to be taken to a mental hospital. So . . . I may need you to shoot me in the head." He knew there were firearms in the house, and in his current state he had little doubt that she would "help" him, so he said it matter-of-factly, like he was asking her to run an errand.

Sofia's eyes widened. Her beloved friend and comrade had just asked her to murder him. But this wise young woman just looked at him, her brow creased with concern, and said, "Why don't you go lie down for a little bit?"

Mollified by this exchange, he went upstairs and lay down on the floor. As he stared at the ceiling, the world began expressing itself in mathematical equations, truths about the nature of reality—staggering in their significance—but he'd dropped out of high school in the 10th grade and none of them made any sense to him.

Over the next couple of hours, the onslaught of thoughts abated, and a sense of normalcy mercifully crept in. His friends returned from the woods, and Sofia informed them about his mental state. They coaxed him downstairs and drove him back to the warehouse in Portland where he lived. He began to realize he was coming back to reality, and a hope dawned in him that things could return to normal. He fell at last into a fitful sleep.

The next day he was shaky. Everything was too bright, too vivid. He thought smoking pot might help—just to take the edge off—but it only triggered another wave of crippling anxiety, terror of a looming mental breakdown. Trembling with fear he waited out the marijuana's effects, unsure if he'd end the night straitjacketed and attempting an unlikely suicide. He walked to the corner store and bought a 40-ounce bottle of malt liquor, grasping for something to still his nerves and get his panic under control.

This set in motion a daily pattern of anxiety, alcohol abuse, and a conviction that madness lurked around every corner. Just hearing the word "schizophrenia" would trigger a full-blown panic attack, and he couldn't be alone for any lengthy period of time. As a panhandler on the Lower East Side of New York City, he developed a habit when he would have to rove the streets alone: asking passersby for the time. His sense of panic would mount toward a breaking point, waves of dizziness and nausea rippling through him, until at last he'd stop and ask a stranger, "Excuse me, do you have the time?" This snippet of social engagement would help settle the roiling inside him, until he walked on and it began to rise again. He found that by asking a person or two on each block for the time he could eventually make it to his destination.

He vowed to never take psychedelics again, and though the squatters and punks in his midst imbibed a rotating diet of intoxicants, he stuck to the alcohol he was convinced would tether him to reality. He was miserable much of the time. And while his previous trauma history likely would have made his transition to adulthood difficult on its own, it did seem that his experimentation with psychedelics had ruined his life.

THE LEATHER CREAKED, HARSH, AND UNCOMFORTABLY LOUD AS the young woman shifted in the therapist's chaise lounge. Her stomach fluttered, which meant either the psilocybin was starting to come on, or she was on the edge of an anxiety attack, or perhaps both. She shifted her body again—another harsh creak.

"Just try to breathe through it," the therapist said.

She had noticed. The therapist had seen her distress. Having a witness brought a sliver of relief. The therapist was older, wise, and a keeper of profound and transformational knowledge.

There was something almost mystical about her, a sage kind of quality. Under her care, everything would be fine, wouldn't it?

The young woman forced in a breath. She'd been looking for a home, a place to belong. She was 25, a psychology graduate student eager for healing. She knew well that she had a stacked deck of trauma to work through. She'd grown up in England and northern Germany, the daughter of a Spanish immigrant who never quite adjusted to German society. Her father, facing constant discrimination, had become angry. His violent outbursts frightened her. Growing up, she looked different from everyone in the Nordic German town. Olive skinned. She felt somehow foreign, even at home. Her mother was a German, the daughter of a fighter pilot—a decorated war hero of the regime, who'd died on the last day of World War II. The shameful, complicated legacy of Nazi Germany had left scars on her family, emotional scars that were too much to process.

The young woman needed a safe place. She needed to know that somewhere, there were people like her with a mixed heritage and conflicted feelings about their upbringings. She traveled the world in search of them, to Asia and Australia to study dance and meditation, looking everywhere for her fellow misfits, searching for deeper meaning and purpose. And this quest for belonging had now brought her across two continents and an ocean, all the way to the west coast of the United States, to the therapist's creaky chaise.

Waves of heat now—colored heat. That had to be the psilocybin. The colors were so bright, so vivid as they unfurled through her mind, opening, changing as the music changed, melding together, interweaving. It was *so beautiful*. She drew a deeper breath.

"Yes, just breathe through it," the therapist said.

She now realized that the interconnected weave of color was

not a mere image but the very substratum of reality, a unifying and loving consciousness that pervaded all things.

She gasped. All of the colors were inextricably linked, inseparable, each an essential strand in the interwoven fabric of the cosmos. And she was one of them. *This* was the feeling of belonging she'd been searching for. It was *here*. It had always been here. She heaved a sigh of relief as a warm wash of awe and wonder flooded her and permeated everything.

But the colors kept changing.

They became even brighter. Too bright. The music climbed to a dizzying crescendo and then crashed down on her, the notes stabbing into her like knives, like chisels into stone, fragmenting her, breaking her apart. Her limbs drew in tight, bound up with terror. Where was the therapist? Where was her guide? She squeezed her eyes shut, waiting for it to end.

It did end, of course. Some days later, she returned to the therapist's office for an integration session. The therapist swiftly dismissed everything she'd experienced: the awe, wonder, and terror. The work was incomplete, she said. The young woman's ego defenses were too thick, and she needed to break through them. She was holding things too tightly, being too sensitive, and too dramatic. Another journey would be necessary, with an even higher dose, and soon.

The young woman slumped in the chair. She felt like a failure. She hesitated to dive back into another journey but trusted this guide. The therapist had seemed like everything she'd been seeking in a mentor: so wise, so worldly, so mature, from a mixed cultural heritage just like herself, and equipped with an exotic array of transformative techniques. She'd trained under shamans from Peru, as well as seasoned Western teachers in the psychedelic underground. It was an impressive lineage, making the young woman trust her. If she needed more psychedelics to break through her ego defenses and get in touch with her innermost nature, then she would take more.

She did more journeys with the therapist, many more. As she delved into her inner depths, she came into contact with her traumatic past. She unearthed the repressed societal shame of the Holocaust, the domestic violence in her family and the existential terror it created, her cultural identity confusion, and her alienation, all bubbling to the surface in that wide-open, vulnerable state, ready for healing and resolution. It was important work, she knew, but it was impossible to contain, all rushing in at once, threatening to break her apart. It was happening far too fast. She needed a protector to help hold it all. She needed someone to see her, to accept her.

"Stop living this trauma story," the therapist often said. "Lots of people have trauma, and yours is nothing special. Just let go." The therapist insisted that she did not need to focus on her familial wounding and its impact on her psyche; she needed to focus on the positive sides of her journeys—the unifying consciousness, the transcendence. Her ego was getting in the way.

Once again, the young woman was doing it wrong. She was a failure. She was unworthy. She became more and more confused about her past. The trauma was her fault, somehow. It was not possible to work through it. She needed to get over it. Her ego defenses were to blame. But her ego defenses were still very much needed to navigate her new immigrant life in the United States. The more she tried to muddle through this haze of conflict and confusion, the more conflicted and confused she became.

Then it was over.

Just like that.

"You need to move on now," the therapist said, ending their relationship.

The young woman was stunned. She'd been given no tools, resources, or way to make sense of what had just happened. All at once, she'd been left with nothing.

Many years of healing work would follow—Hakomi, Somatic Experiencing (SE), Continuum, embodied meditation—all with qualified and compassionate practitioners. As the young woman went inside, she found again and again that she was not only working through the trauma of her childhood but the damage inflicted by her psychedelic therapist. She'd been given mind-opening drugs in the context of a relationship that was fundamentally unsafe and then been abandoned by her provider without warning. And while she'd approached every psilocybin journey eager for healing and integration, her therapist—with years of professional experience and a booming private practice—had only left her with more trauma and fragmentation.

THESE ARE OUR STORIES. JOSHUA AND MANUELA.

We offer them to you as cautionary tales. Let's be crystal clear about this from the start: Danger is inherent to the use of psychedelics. Although we write this book to affirm and celebrate their potential value as medicines, we must also recognize that these powerful drugs can create significant psychological damage. We want to do everything we can to ensure that psychedelics are used in therapeutic ways, maximizing their value for growth and change. For we are that teenage revolutionary looking for liberation, that mid-twenties seeker on her path of transformation, and we now find ourselves as *wounded healers* supporting the growth and healing of our students and clients. We want psychedelic therapy to truly *work* for those who yearn for greater ease and fulfillment in their lives.

For this to happen, it is essential to understand the role of the facilitator, guide, or sitter who accompanies the person on psychedelics. A general rule of thumb is that people shouldn't take these medicines alone, especially if they are looking for a therapeutic experience. In Indigenous traditions that work with consciousness-altering plants, a shaman often guides the process. They have usually completed a decades-long apprenticeship, acquainting themselves with the medicine before administering it to others, carriers of an ancient tradition reflecting generations of learning and accumulated wisdom.

In cultures lacking these traditional practices—such as the modern West—other ways of creating guardrails for the psychedelic experience have been developed. Some communities of recreational users describe the importance of a *tripsitter* (sometimes shortened to *sitter*), a sober peer who makes sure the person on the trip is OK. The sitter is not necessarily there to do therapy, but is necessary for *harm reduction*. It's recognized that getting high on these drugs requires a clearheaded companion.

Still others describe the person providing accompaniment as a "facilitator." This term may emphasize that the goal is not to make something happen but simply to hold space and allow a process to unfold. A facilitator often has more training than a sitter, and sometimes prepares the journeyer beforehand and assists them in integrating the experience afterward. Some facilitators are also mental health professionals. Both licensed psychotherapists and other facilitators may have completed long apprenticeships and/or rigorous training programs in psychedelic-assisted therapy.

Yet another role is that of the *prescriber*, a physician or psychiatrist who dispenses controlled substances. Some medicines used in psychedelic-assisted therapy require a medical professional's prescription to access. Different countries and states—as well as counties or municipalities within those states—have different laws. Some clients will be interacting with multiple professionals as they seek care.

However they are described, there should be another person there to support the process. We primarily use the term "therapist" to describe this role, though this is not meant to indicate that only licensed mental health professionals can do this work. Whether you prefer the term "sitter," "facilitator," or "therapist," we know that the potential value in taking a psychedelic is greatly enhanced when the user has someone with them, particularly if that person is trusted and has the ability to pay attention, support what emerges, and contain the experience. This book is our attempt to give the best guidance possible to anyone who wants to assist a person on psychedelics to get the maximal benefit from their journey.

These medicines are powerful shapers and changers of consciousness, often bringing up unexpected material with a strong emotional charge. Such dramatically altered perception is often challenging, especially for people accustomed to regularity and predictability in their day-to-day lives. The anarchic or *high entropy* cognition of psychedelics can feel distressing for those who equate safety with control over their thoughts and feelings. Drugs that disrupt the normal flow of conscious experience can engender a sense of powerlessness for some people, a feeling of suspended agency and acute vulnerability. For this reason, having someone there who can look out for danger is vital. On a bodily level, we may need another human in close proximity to help us relinquish our accustomed vigilance and allow things to unfold.

Besides attending to the user (we mostly use the term "journeyer" to describe this individual), the trained psychedelic therapist knows when to say or do particular things that will increase the probability of a therapeutic outcome. Psychedelics can bring incredible insights, allowing the unconscious to penetrate into awareness and lay bare our unfinished business. These truths can feel monumental and incredibly profound, but such transcendent illumination is meaningless if one is unable to integrate the experience and make use of it. Whether we prefer to think of the psychedelic journey as a therapeutic process or a spiritual rite, it must have guardrails around it to protect the safety of the journeyer, allowing them to assimilate the journey and change afterward. Without a solid container for the work and a path for processing it afterward, it is worth questioning whether psychedelics should be taken at all.

Both of us completed a rigorous training program to become certified in psychedelic-assisted therapy (as well as methylenedioxymethamphetamine [MDMA]-assisted therapy). While we learned a great deal from these trainings, as well as from our own experiences and from research into the state of this field, it became clear that a book outlining the best practices for psychedelic-assisted somatic therapists was sorely needed. Our professional experience supporting journeys and helping people recover from the trauma of "bad trips" has given us a healthy respect for these medicines. As mindfulness practitioners, psychotherapists, and teachers of somatic and trauma-treatment modalities for decades, we've been able to survey various healing traditions and build a coherent body of theory and practice. Our hope is that elucidating this will be of benefit to the field of psychedelic therapy.

We should mention that we are not doctors, and nothing in this book is meant to constitute medical advice. We strongly advise anyone interested in this topic to consult medical professionals before making any decisions that could impact their health—or that of others.

THERE IS CURRENTLY A STRONG BIAS TOWARD MENTATION (MENtal activity) in psychedelic work. The name "psychedelic" itself betrays this, the Greek word form signifying something that is *mind manifesting*. While some would argue that a more faithful translation would be soul *manifesting*, modern English speakers generally conflate *psyche* with mind rather than soul. This is congruent with Western culture's fixation on cognitive processing, an entrenched way of life that is overly identified with thoughts, where the location of the self is somewhere behind one's eyes. As René Descartes—one of the most influential thinkers in all of Western philosophy—put it: "I think, therefore I am." In the Western world, existence itself is equated with thinking. We in the West are the inheritors of a disembodied and abstracted mode of being that denies any significant role for nature or the human body.

Throughout this book we argue that psychedelics are also *body manifesting* (or *somadelic*) in their mode of action, subjective effects, and enduring impact on the journeyer's life. As teachers of body-centered psychotherapy, we are heartened to see that the greater psychedelic space seems open to somatic practices. But for this to have any meaningful impact, therapists must possess a skillful, nuanced understanding of how to work with the body to support an *embodied journey*.

MANUELA IS A SENIOR TRAINER AT THE HAKOMI INSTITUTE, teaching the Hakomi approach to healing developed by Ron Kurtz. Joshua is a faculty member at Somatic Experiencing International, leading professional trainings in the Somatic Experiencing® (or, SE™) methodology originated by Peter Levine, PhD.* While there are differences between the two, both Hakomi

---

* The views, opinions, methodologies, and practices that Joshua expresses or recommends in this book are his own and do not necessarily reflect the official views of SEI. SEI does not endorse, approve, or support any specific authors, practitioners, or contributors unless explicitly stated otherwise.

and SE incorporate body awareness to support the innate healing impulse in each of us—what Stanislav Grof (2006) called the *inner healing intelligence*. Levine (1997) describes SE as "a naturalistic approach" (p. 6), while Hakomi explicitly identifies organicity as one of five core principles (Kurtz, 2015). In other words, both approaches work in a way that is *bottom-up*, inviting the unconscious, embodied aspect of our experience into healing. This stands in stark relief with the current state of psychotherapy, which focuses more on thoughts and *top-down* control.

If you've taken psychedelics, you've seen firsthand that top-down control is often inaccessible. This is one reason we're excited to bring our decades of teaching and clinical experience in the field of somatics to psychedelic therapy, offering practitioners the necessary skills to facilitate a bottom-up therapeutic process.

Another reason we're excited to collaborate on this book is that it represents a synthesis of insights from both SE and Hakomi. For too long, division has dominated the therapeutic world, with various theoreticians coming forward to claim terrain in a capitalistic landscape. Separating into divergent modalities at times reflects significant differences in approach, but often seems purely profit driven—a ploy to corner the market and gain stature rather than serve the healing of the world. With this book we are committing to a higher truth than the alleged superiority of particular modalities, breaking down unnecessary divisions in service of more expansion and greater organization for those we serve. These goals, of course, are wholly congruent with the insights achieved in many psychedelic journeys, something that is not lost on us.

This cultural moment—including the promising new direction of psychedelic-assisted therapy—is a leap forward in the field of psychological science, one that holds immense promise for change. If psychedelic therapy is held well it can be a safe and effective way to heal trauma, treat certain kinds of psychopathology, aid in what's been called the *betterment of well people*, and potentially even help to change the culture at large. Our world is desperately in need of this change, as existential threats loom more menacing every day.

If the journeyer can return from the expansive inner world of the psychedelic experience bearing the treasures offered there, it is possible that our world can be transformed to more closely resemble that one. Many people report that psychedelics teach them—often after an arduous trial of renegotiating personal traumas—that the beings of this world are interconnected, that at our core we all want to live with goodwill, and that fear is a corrosive influence that poisons the well of our collective psyche. These insights are desperately needed as guideposts at this critical time of ecological crisis and political instability. We should safeguard any pathway through which such wisdom can arise and be integrated into our culture. This is our ultimate goal. Let us endeavor to become as good as we can possibly be at holding space for the psychedelic experience, knowing that when individuals heal they also impact the collective.

EMBODIED PSYCHEDELIC THERAPY

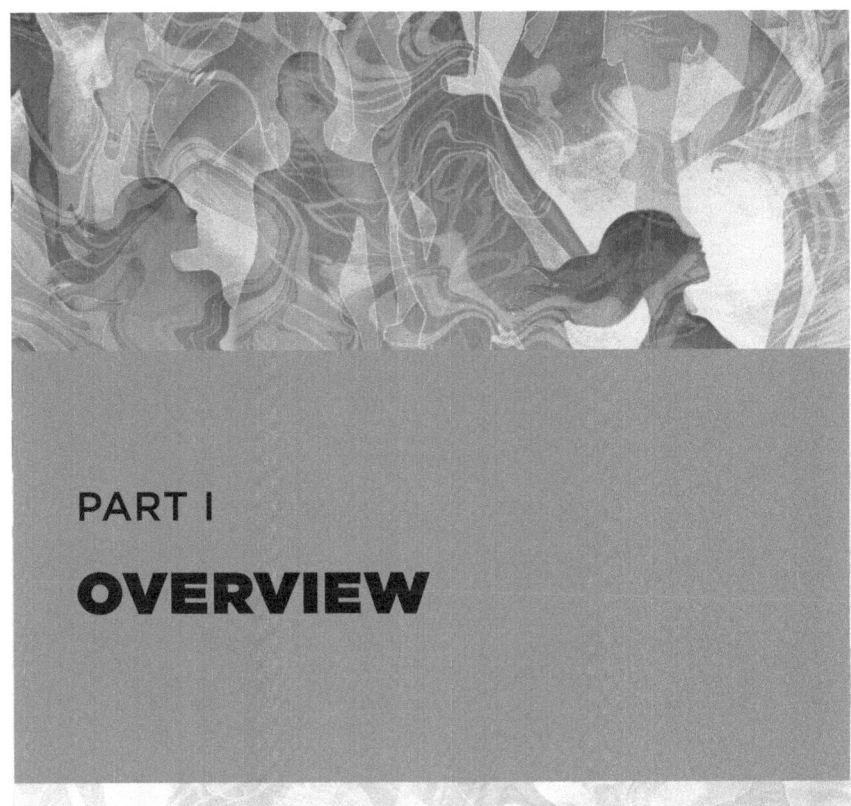

PART I
OVERVIEW

CHAPTER 1

The Field of Psychedelic Therapy

> *"The potential significance of . . . psychedelics for psychiatry and psychology [is] comparable to the value the microscope has for biology and medicine or the telescope has for astronomy."*
> —STANISLAV GROF

It has been said that Western culture is in the midst of a "psychedelic renaissance," a paradigm shift in how people think about therapy involving consciousness-expanding drugs. European and North American scientists first discovered these medicines in the late 1890s (e.g., Ellis, 1898), though they'd been used for millennia in Indigenous societies. In the 20th century they were celebrated as catalysts for therapeutic change. Experimenters in that era performed rigorous studies proving their efficacy in treating a wide range of psychological maladies.

In fact, over 1,000 scientific papers (documenting over 40,000 participants) were authored in the 1950s and 1960s on the use of psychedelics for treating various conditions (Grinspoon & Balakar, 1979). But when these substances escaped the lab, splashing into the youth counterculture of the late 1960s, the resultant revolution in consciousness threatened the status quo, generating a backlash of epic proportions. As psychedelics were outlawed and vilified, the Western world came to see them as inherently dangerous—perhaps even *evil*—with lurid stories of suicide and descents into madness splashed across the covers of magazines and newspapers. For a time, the therapeutic potential of the psychedelic experience seemed to be lost forever.

In the 1990s, courageous experimenters began to undertake carefully controlled studies of psychedelics again, with regulatory agencies exerting tremendous pressure from above. The stigma surrounding altered states of consciousness made it difficult for these scientists to get their research approved, but privately funded charities like the Multidisciplinary Association for Psychedelic Studies (MAPS) provided them with crucial support. New data emerged, kindling a hope that the skillful incorporation of psychedelics into psychiatry was possible. It's probably not an accident that this occurred at a time when interest in conventional psychiatric medications was on the wane. The antidepressant and antipsychotic drugs that once held so much promise were recognized as weak and inconsistent treatments (Healy, 1997; Kirsch & Sapirstein, 1998).

There now exists clear empirical evidence that psychedelics change people's lives. Critically, though, these experiments show efficacy for psychedelic-assisted *therapy*. Each paper details how researchers conducted multiple preparation sessions before administering the drug, and followed the experience with multiple integration sessions. In the MAPS protocol (Mithoefer, 2016), for instance, posttraumatic stress disorder (PTSD) sufferers are given three preparation sessions before their first dose of MDMA, with each preparation session lasting 60–90 minutes. After each of the three MDMA experiences, three lengthy integration sessions occur. In other words, there is extensive preparation for the drug experience, and integration work following—a minimum of 12 hours of intensive therapy in addition to the time spent under the influence of the drug. In a paper published in the *Journal of Psychopharmacology*, MAPS researchers Michael and Annie

Mithoefer (and colleagues; 2011) describe MDMA as a "catalyst to psychotherapy" (p. 440). It is clear that they are not studying drug effects per se but rather how drugs can be utilized in the context of therapy. In other words, *the science behind the psychedelic renaissance is about therapy, not just the drugs themselves.*

TRAINING FOR PSYCHEDELIC THERAPISTS

The education of psychedelic therapists matters. Experiential training preparing them to hold space for journeyers—before, during, and after the drug experience—is key to good outcomes. As well, it's crucial to maintaining momentum for psychedelic work. If these medicines are finally legalized (or even rescheduled), only to fall into the hands of poorly trained facilitators unequipped to support the journey, it could spell disaster. We believe modern journeyers require a competent therapist or guide if the goal is to achieve stable, long-term behavioral change.

PSYCHEDELICS FOR WEIRD PEOPLE

As mentioned, many traditional cultures utilize consciousness-altering substances. There is archeological and anthropological evidence for psychedelic use going back into prehistory, and Indigenous societies have developed wise practices to support journeyers in expanded states. We honor and celebrate these traditions, seeing them as wholly valid ways to support an embodied journey, and would never suggest that a member of such societies needs a guide trained in Western therapy.

These catalysts for healing have been used in ceremonial contexts for thousands of years. Humans around the world pursue expanded states of consciousness for healing, to connect with ancestors, engage with the spirits of plants and animals (as well as other deities), and to attain wisdom. In an earth-based culture attuned to the rhythms of nature, with a pantheistic psychospiritual worldview, entering into psychedelic states is likely easy to integrate. The altered state is not so different from trance regularly accessed through immersion in wilderness, mythic storytelling at the fireside, and rites of initiation involving fasting or the transmogrification of the flesh.

Individuals from Western, educated, industrialized, rich, and democratic (WEIRD) countries (Henrich et al., 2010), however, receive none of this preparation. They often have no exposure to coherent worldviews that could help one make sense of the psychedelic experience. Trained to rely on the intellect, it could be terrifying to feel one's rationality slipping away. Taught to maintain control over one's emotions, it could be extremely threatening when feelings come unbidden to the surface. Inculcated into scientific materialism, it could be bewildering to be suddenly thrust into animism.

Because Westerners lack the cultural frameworks to prepare for, hold, and integrate the psychedelic journey, it is incumbent on the therapist to provide an adequate proxy. In our preparation sessions, we answer questions and offer guidance to make the experience safer. During the journey, we lovingly—but unsentimentally—hold space for what unfolds. In the integration phase, we reinforce the journeyer's innate wisdom.

There have been, in the modern, Western world, underground communities that carried on psychedelic therapy even after it was outlawed. When legitimate research and legal practice were suddenly criminalized, a network of helpers refused to bow to unconscionable prohibitions. In these communities, one would have been exposed to models of the world that—in a way similar to the indigenous cultures mentioned above—prepared them to usefully integrate psychedelic work.

Prospective journeyers in the modern West lack a cultural container for psychedelics, a lineage of practice for gestating and integrating what gets revealed. It is therefore necessary to generate well-trained and competent therapists who can hold these powerful experiences, particularly at this critical juncture in Western culture's relationship with psychedelics. It is worth remembering, again, that protocols proving efficacy for psychedelic-assisted therapy involve multiple nondrug sessions, and always include at least one therapist present for the entirety of any dosing session. In other words, *the science behind the psychedelic renaissance is about therapists, not just the drugs themselves.*

PSYCHEDELICS AND PSYCHIATRY

As psychedelics continue to be woven into mainstream psychiatry, we must ensure that the central role of the therapist is understood. Psychopharmacology—administering drugs to alter the neurological underpinnings of conscious states—generally pursues *psychotropic cures.* Thus far, the field has been biased toward a disease model, where mental suffering is seen as a disordered biological process correctable via mechanistic means.

Psychiatry says that a struggling patient simply needs a doctor to prescribe the right medicine to treat their neurological imbalances. However, there are clear data that patients show greater improvement from a combination of pharmaceuticals *and* therapy than from drugs alone (Cuijpers et al., 2015). Alleviating suffering through the daily dosing of chemicals leaves the underlying issue untreated.

An effort to eliminate pain—to make it disappear—is a fool's errand. In fact, the distress that motivates people to seek psychiatric help provides an opportunity for healing—to loosen psychic knots, integrate previously unassimilable experiences, and come more fully into alignment with one's true self. Psychology has often sought to make people more *well-adjusted*—or better able to function in society—but adjustment should never be the sole goal of therapy. Therapists should support people to come fully into themselves, in body and mind, growing into their own idiosyncratic wisdom. We believe that psychological science can relinquish its mission to make an enemy of anxiety, depression, addiction, PTSD, and other disorders.

Psychedelics represent an opposite approach. The psychedelic experience often brings a person's core wounds vividly to light, producing insights that open the possibility of new ways of being. As patients let go of the Sisyphean task of pushing distress away, they discover a freedom and completeness they never thought possible. Indeed, a significant healing power of psychedelics is the self-acceptance they make possible. Psychedelics often compel people to turn *toward* their distress, allowing them to see the underlying forces that keep them stuck in maladaptive patterns. The psychedelic renaissance promises a sea change in our culture's approach to treating mental pain, moving us away from a simplistic wish to escape suffering and toward a more mature willingness to work through what ails us.

THE MODERN ERA OF PSYCHEDELICS

Studies indicate that psychedelic-assisted therapy is effective for depression (Davis et al., 2021), end-of-life distress (Yu et al., 2021), addictions (van der Meer et al., 2023), PTSD (Mitchell et al., 2023), and other maladies. This is a boon for sufferers, especially those who may not have responded well to conventional treatments. However, psychedelics can also support people without a diagnosis to feel better and more fulfilled. We have seen time and again how a skillfully guided psychedelic experience can benefit people without diagnosed mental health disorders. They may discover a deeper purpose in their life, renew their sense of connection to others, and access truths they'd been avoiding. We don't think psychedelics should be reserved for treating psychopathology, with the medicine being prescribed to "fix" people. We hope for a future in which the psychedelic experience is available as a resource for anyone aspiring to know themselves better, live with more authenticity and ease, and recover their sense of meaning.

However, psychedelics are not a panacea, and we should avoid idealizing these substances or the altered state they produce. Some popularizers of psychedelics seem afflicted with a rosy-eyed mysticism, which may hinder our efforts to make these medicines more widely available. Let's not forget that only a few decades ago, stoned Utopians schemed about putting LSD in the water, convinced that deliverance for all was only a dose away.

In the rush to commodify psychedelics, business interests are making claims that are too good to be true. They may end up repeating failed psychiatric fads of the past, where a new drug gets marketed with outrageous claims about its effectiveness, a corporation cashes in, and a couple decades later everyone realizes it didn't do what it was purported to.

Psychedelics don't work for everyone. Some find them unpleasant or overwhelming, while others find them colorful and vivid but not conducive to growth or healing. Even if the journey itself is therapeutic, the journeyer still must integrate what emerges. While psychedelics can reveal things to us, it is not guaranteed that our lives will change as a result.

There are also contraindications for psychedelics, situations in which they are not the optimal treatment (or would require great care and consideration). In the famous studies that ignited the psychedelic renaissance, not just anyone was allowed to be a subject (e.g., Carhart-Harris et al., 2016). There were clear rule outs:

Some applicants were told in the assessment phase they weren't good candidates. This included anyone with a history of psychosis, or who had a first-order relative with schizophrenia or bipolar disorder. Were this safeguard not in place, there almost certainly would have been more adverse events and bad outcomes, and the resultant data would be far less compelling. We need to carefully screen potential journeyers to ensure we don't give psychedelics to vulnerable individuals who may not receive their benefits—or worse, could be harmed by them.

HOW DO PSYCHEDELICS WORK?

How do psychedelics work? Many theories exist about their mechanism of action, several of which revolve around the brain.

Robin Carhart-Harris, founder and former lead of the Centre for Psychedelic Research at Imperial College London (now in the Department of Neurology at the University of California, San Francisco [UCSF]), has published influential research on the brain's response to psychedelics. He was the lead author for multiple studies on the efficacy of psilocybin for treatment-resistant depression (Carhart-Harris et al., 2016), using functional magnetic resonance imaging (fMRI) data to demonstrate how psychedelics change the brain in unusual ways (Carhart-Harris et al., 2017).

Psychedelics create a condition Carhart-Harris termed the "anarchic brain" (Carhart-Harris & Friston, 2019; he later adopted the phrase "entropic brain"). The disruption of overdetermined neurological patterns—automatic, repetitive mental states that can give rise to the symptoms of psychopathology—is a major feature of the psychedelic journey. His findings show that brains are more malleable during and after psychedelic experiences, creating a precious opportunity for shifts in perspective and self-understanding. These *windows of neuroplasticity*—transitory periods when neural pathways can be rewired—shift the way our brains process information and respond to the environment. In day-to-day life, changing our habitual responses is very difficult, leaving us stuck in conditioned patterns that may be unsatisfying. Interrupting this creates opportunities to break out of the prison of self-defeating routines.

Carhart-Harris and colleagues (2023) borrow a term from genetics to describe the fixity typifying much of day-to-day life: "canalization." According to *Hebb's Law*—a cornerstone of neuroscience—neurons that fire together, wire together (Hebb, 1949). Once the neural network in our brain crystallizes, our thinking and behavior tend to recur in the same ways, over and over again. This is not unlike the canals that cut through seaside cities, permitting only one route between two points—hence *canalization*. Psychedelics allow for *de-canalization*, where neurological patterns of fixity are temporarily loosened and new connections are possible.

In a related analogy, Michael Pollan (2018)—bestselling author and advocate of psychedelic therapy—compares the mind to a ski slope. As we ski downhill we create deeper and deeper grooves in the snow, and with each descent we become more and more likely to follow these paths. Psychedelics act as the "snow groomer," clearing away these grooves and allowing the skier to trace a new route on the next descent. Should this new pathway prove more rewarding, it can then be followed in subsequent runs. In other words, psychedelics allow more adaptive patterns of thought and behavior to emerge. So, one aspect of the anarchic brain is that it is less bound by habitual forces, making us freer.

Another aspect of the anarchic brain is that it is more interconnected. Neuroimaging data have demonstrated that psychedelics allow far-flung parts of the brain to communicate with one another more easily (Daws et al., 2022), allowing novel insights to emerge that can change brain function in enduring ways. This is related to the brain's *modularity*.

Over the previous century, neuroscience has shown that the brain is a modular system, where particular brain regions are responsible for specific functions. Put different people in a brain imaging machine and ask them to complete an exercise—you will see a specific region consistently light up on the scans. The brightness on the scan represents increased blood flow, and hence, activity. For instance, we have certain areas (*modules*) involved in recognizing faces (*fusiform face area*), decoding speech (*Wernicke's area*), producing speech (*Broca's area*), and so on. This understanding has helped delineate the different specializations of the two brain hemispheres, and has identified three distinct neurological structures: the brainstem and cerebellum (involved in maintaining bodily homeostasis), the limbic system (responsible for emotion processing), and the cortex (performing higher-order abstract cognitive functions). These different hemispheres, levels, and modules do communicate with one another, but in day-to-day functioning they tend to keep more to their own neurological neighborhoods. During psychedelic experiences, however, communication pathways between modules are opened, creating more chaotic internetworking and novel collaborative neurological function.

Yet another aspect of the anarchic brain is that *downstream processing* is liberated, allowing it to emerge more easily into consciousness. Usually, a tremendous amount of mental processing occurs below the threshold of awareness, or *downstream*, as the brain automates necessary functions and carefully limits what emerges into conscious attention. Psychedelics flood the brain with molecules that bind to particular receptor sites, disrupting the usual filtering of more primitive brain processes. As a result, the journeyer receives more direct information about their moment-to-moment experience and is less encumbered by preconceived conceptual frameworks, seeing and understanding things in new ways. Journeyers may discover new perspectives, with some remarking on a sense of familiarity to the insights they discover. We regularly hear things like "I now know it's true. On some level, I knew it already, but I just didn't *know* that I knew it." Carhart-Harris and colleagues call this style of *bottom-up* information processing RElaxed Beliefs Under pSychedelics (REBUS; Carhart-Harris & Friston, 2019). As brain processes that are usually unconscious emerge into awareness, the relaxation of prior beliefs allows us to consider things anew.

So, the anarchic brain is (a) less constrained by prior habits, (b) more interconnected, and (c) less centralized and more democratic. Lower brain regions communicate more with the higher, there is a generalized lack of separateness that allows parts of the brain to talk to one another more easily, and brain networks don't follow the same well-trodden paths over and over. These conditions create neuroplasticity, real-time alterations in brain function that facilitate change.

THE IMPORTANCE OF THE BODY

That's a lot about the brain, but what about the rest of the body? While the neurobiological model can help us understand the psychedelic's powerful effects on thinking and feeling, we don't think it tells the whole story.

Theorists sometimes describe the embodied aspect of psychedelics as peripheral to the main event. As with many things in Western culture, this dismissive view emphasizes the abstract, cognitive aspect of the experience. Books on psychedelic therapy discuss "body load," a superficial sensory experience that they seem to fear could distract journeyers from the real work. But the change process in psychedelic therapy intrinsically involves the body.

On psychedelics, our body discharges pent-up energy, enacts incomplete motor impulses, expresses emotions and insights through patterned movement, and in many ways drives the process of transformation. Journeyers describe feeling "lighter," a sense of "flow," or that something has been "lifted" from them. Parts of the body may feel "heavy," or they may feel "tightness," or that there is an energy dwelling in certain parts of the body. *These are not just metaphors.* The body and brain are in constant communication. In fact, the field of *embodied cognition* has come to recognize that what we often take to be abstract psychological states are deterministically influenced by bodily state. The power of psychedelics to "loosen psychic knots" mentioned earlier will also, by necessity, mean a loosening of physical knots. The body and brain are an indissoluble unity, and one needs to skillfully work with the body in psychedelic therapy to achieve the desired outcome.

Many approaches to psychedelic therapy suggest that the journeyer should lie still throughout the experience, with some even claiming that physical movement would be somehow counterfeit. Spontaneous discharge of energy in the body is seen as a distraction, rather than an essential driver of the openness necessary for neuroplasticity. In this book, we emphasize the importance of giving attention to the body, recognizing its "voice," and supporting what wants to emerge at the level of sensorimotor processing.

SUPPORT FOR BOTTOM-UP PROCESSING

Throughout this book we describe the practices we think psychedelic therapists need to know. At this point, though, we want to offer a quick word on the fundamental attitude that best supports psychedelic therapy and integration.

As mentioned in the Introduction, the Somatic Experiencing methodology offers a naturalistic approach (Levine, 1997), and Hakomi focuses on organicity as a core principle (Kurtz, 2015). This is because—in contradistinction to the precepts of industrial civilization—the human organism is a self-healing psychophysiological entity. The body knows how to knit together wounded flesh and generate a scar to bridge the gap, provided that we do two things: clean the wound to prevent infection and bandage the area to protect it from further injury. Similarly, the deep structure of the psyche knows how to rectify damage to its integrity. If we create the right conditions, the mind will administer its own healing and transformation.

For this reason, we think the most important task of the therapist (psychedelic or otherwise) is to ally ourselves with the inner healing intelligence of the client, resisting the impulse to superimpose our own ideas about what should happen or attempt to control the process. This *nondirective* approach has been highlighted in the world of psychedelic therapy, with many writers emphasizing the importance of therapists not getting in the way. However, we've noticed a curious tendency for researchers and theoreticians to give explicit instruction that therapists be nondirective, on the one hand, while implicitly modeling directive interventions, on the other. This is very confusing! Many trainees in psychedelic therapy programs have come to us trying to understand why it was hammered into them to be nondirective, while at the same time their instructors emphasized therapist technique. Many have reported watching demonstrations that involved a huge amount of intervention on the part of the therapist, which contravened the mantra of being nondirective.

It is true that much of being a good psychedelic therapist involves being able to *do nothing* (or at least seem to be doing nothing). That said, the therapist's presence is key to a good outcome, and it is crucial we know what to do in those moments when it's necessary to intervene. Much of this book is a guide on how to *be* with someone on psychedelics (or integrating a psychedelic experience afterward), rather than a primer on what to *do* in the presence of a journeyer. This will produce the most therapeutic results, giving journeyers a sense that they did something for themselves—rather than something having been done *to* them, or *for* them. We trust that when therapists absorb this principle, it benefits not just those they serve but also their own unfolding as a person.

CHAPTER 2

The Centrality of Ethics

Mature revelation demands mature people . . . mature people vitalize culture through their individual and collective actions.
—BILL PLOTKIN

THE IMPACT OF ETHICS VIOLATIONS

MDMA-assisted therapy (MDMA-AT) for the treatment of PTSD has been around for decades, and rigorously studied since the early 2010s (Mithoefer et al., 2011), yet it continues to languish in the Food and Drug Administration (FDA) approval process. Concerns have been raised about MDMA researchers' unethical approach to data collection—pressuring study participants to report only positive results—as well as their sexual misconduct and boundary violations (Mustafa et al., 2024). Mounting evidence from clinical trials, as well as reams of anecdotal data, indicate its efficacy. However, partly because the research process has been marred by ethical transgressions, approval has been delayed unnecessarily. This serves as a sobering reminder of the centrality of ethical conduct in psychedelic therapy and research.

Let's be clear: Psychedelics initiate significant shifts in consciousness, but this is not an inherent good. These drugs can be utilized for healing and transformation, but they can also be tools of exploitation in the hands of unethical actors. The Central Intelligence Agency's (CIA's) Project MKUltra program is an infamous example. The CIA was actually the largest funder of LSD research in the 1950s (Lee & Shlain, 1992), as they sought to develop a truth serum to be used on prisoners of war and suspected agents of espionage. Unwitting subjects were psychologically tortured in the CIA's experiments, and there were several deaths.

We can also look back on the crimes of the Manson Family. Using isolation, obligatory orgies, and frequent acid trips to soften the minds of his followers, "Charlie" proselytized about the coming race war and his messianic aspirations. In fact, his use of LSD to increase the suggestibility of Family members may have come directly from MKUltra operatives (O'Neill, 2019). The murders committed in Manson's name attest to the value-neutral quality of psychedelics. We shouldn't assume that "the medicine" is inherently healing, or intrinsically *good*. If given in the wrong context, it can ruin a person's life, or even end it.

ETHICS AND PSYCHEDELICS

Any healer worth the name should devote themselves to ethics, as this determines what's possible for those they serve. If our ethical commitment is lax, clients can be harmed. On the other hand, if we're overly rigid in our adherence to abstract rules, we may not meet our clients on a human level, thereby failing to support their unique healing process.

Many laws and ethical codes now govern the practice of psychotherapy, but this wasn't always the case. In the late 19th century, hypnotherapists began using the "talking cure" without any regulatory oversight. Absurdly unethical behavior ensued, and some patients came away emotionally damaged. This slowly gave way to regulation, with boards and agencies legislating minimum standards of care for consumers.

Today, licensed professionals must abide by a long list of guidelines. On top of legal restrictions, one's professional memberships may involve additional sets of regulations. This is necessary, as it protects clients from abuse and substandard care.

Psychedelic-assisted therapy presents further challenges to the ethical delivery of care than does traditional psychotherapy. Those working with expanded states of consciousness need to commit to ethical precepts, adopting practices to minimize harm *before* working with people. This is a precondition for a healing therapeutic relationship.

Psychedelic work differs from other therapies—the journeyer *is* intoxicated, after all. Clients are in a highly dependent, vulnerable mental state: whether considering psychedelic work, in the middle of a journey, or integrating it afterward. People on psychedelics are also suggestible. The mind is more porous, the ego less defended. The things a therapist says or does—or doesn't say or do—can be exceptionally impactful. Journeyers may be subject to the whims of the guide, relinquishing their autonomy and capacity for critical thinking.

A not uncommon feature of psychedelic trips is *regression*, when a full-grown adult may find themselves feeling childlike. Like children everywhere, they are susceptible to seeing the authority in the room—in this case, the therapist—as *right* and their own intuitions as *wrong*. They may see the therapist as the ultimate arbiter of truth.

The therapist, though, is also touched by the altered state. The phenomenon of the "contact high" is well-known—being in a room with someone on drugs will alter the consciousness of the sober person. In this heady space, relational challenges sometimes arise. Therapeutic dynamics—complex under normal circumstances—are intensified in psychedelic work. Grof (1980) called LSD a "powerful unspecific amplifier or catalyst of . . . neurophysiological processes in the brain" (p. 52). Psychedelics amplify mental processes; also amplified is the intensity of the relationship between therapist and client. Our preconceived assumptions about our role may suddenly come into question. Therefore, an ironclad commitment to ethical precepts will serve us well in this nonordinary space.

Ethics can be counterintuitive. It is often challenging to translate one's intent to help others into skillful therapeutic presence. As healers, we must develop a new set of assumptions about relating. We have each been conditioned into automatic ways of responding to people, but these can interfere with the therapeutic relationship.

There are also many ethical considerations specific to psychedelic-assisted therapy. One of these is that we should acknowledge teachers and the source of much of our knowledge. Indigenous groups have practiced these approaches for a long, long time. There is a danger in the Western psychedelic renaissance of seeing this work as "innovative," or "groundbreaking," but it's simply a recycling of the social technology our ancestors have always known. The current rush to commodify psychedelics may end up hurting the communities that have safeguarded them for millennia—with ayahuasca tourism, neo-shamanism, the overharvest of peyote, and various kinds of cultural appropriation degrading the traditions that should be uplifted. It is one of our responsibilities as psychedelic therapists to make sure indigenous voices are heard. Ethically, we need to ensure that the medicalization of psychedelics doesn't omit the perspectives of earth-based cultures. The entire field owes a debt to the longtime keepers of psychedelic wisdom traditions around the world.

CODES OF ETHICS

There is at present no widely adopted ethical code for psychedelic-assisted therapy. However, there have been efforts to redress this gap. MAPS (2021) has their *Code of Ethics*, and the American Psychedelic Practitioners Association (APPA; 2023) published *Professional Practice Guidelines*. In Oregon, where psilocybin-assisted therapy is regulated, facilitators agree to the *Ethical Principles/Code of Conduct* issued by the Oregon Health Authority (OHA; 2022).

Licensed physicians and psychotherapists have their own codes to abide by, but these may not cover the exigencies demanded by psychedelic work. One should always be aware of the most restrictive code governing particular choices. For instance, healthy touch with consent is generally considered ethical in psychedelic therapy, but certain mental health professionals are prohibited from making physical contact. In these instances, we need to carefully weigh our ethical obligations to institutions against the needs of our clients and patients.

Also, the field of psychedelic-assisted therapy is new and rapidly developing. Original research emerges constantly—exploring variations in dosage, documenting adverse events, and in other ways facilitating new perspectives on the practice. A commitment to ethical work requires that we stay abreast of new developments in the field.

OUTER ETHICS AND INNER ETHICS

We are each required to ratify our commitment to specific ethical codes in our chosen field, but unethical behavior does not simply disappear when legislated against. Institutions impose penalties for the violation of behavioral norms, which may be a necessity in complex societies. We should encourage helpers to *want* to behave ethically, though, based on accumulated wisdom about what helps (or hurts) those we serve. In other words, ethics are best understood as principles or values that we hold—and the study of how we channel those into action—rather than rules or mores that are arbitrarily imposed upon us.

Kylea Taylor (2017) invokes a helpful model for this, differentiating between outer and inner ethics. *Outer ethics* are the commonsensical notions given in our professions, codified as rules and regulations. These can be important guideposts along the way. *Inner ethics*, on the other hand, are our own convictions about what is *right* or *good*. These may differ from the received values of our community, mentors, or professional organization. We need to take time to inquire into our personal relationship with ethics. What promises will we make to ourselves as we take on the sacred task of helping others heal?

As with everything else, this involves the body. We often speak of what's "in our gut," an instinctive knowing that hews to the truth. We also refer to what we know "in our heart," a core intuition more real than the thinking mind. We can learn a lot about thorny ethical dilemmas simply by paying attention to our bodies, cutting through the rationalizations and justifications the ego expertly devises to get what it wants.

The psychedelic therapist must compassionately interrogate their own motives and actions, recognizing how normal processes of ethical slippage can be intensified in psychedelic therapy. Simply put, we may not be in command of our normal faculties. We need to make preemptive pledges about how we'll act in our professional role.

During the session, and afterward, we should be curious about the impulses that arise—those we acted on, and those we didn't— bringing gentle curiosity as to why we were impelled in these ways.

These investigations can begin to bring our shadow into the light of consciousness.

Try This: What Is My Relationship to Ethics?

Take a moment and consider the word *ethics*. What associations arise? Does this word evoke coercion, a feeling of being forced into something? Or is there a sense of connecting more deeply to yourself, freeing your own conviction to be who you truly are? Drop your awareness into your body . . . does it constrict when you hear this word? Does it relax? Get warm? Cold?

Take a break and attend to these sensations, trying not to judge your experience. See if there are any shifts, and if these shifts inform your relationship to the word "ethics."

Now, remember a time when you faced a difficult choice between getting something you wanted and honoring your own sense of who you really are. When did you make the hard choice to do the right thing? How do you feel about that choice now? What happens in your body as you think about this? How does this incline you to act in the future?

BOUNDARY VIOLATIONS

Psychedelic therapy needs ethics. These drugs inherently involve crossing thresholds, breaking through limitations, and reinventing reality. Journeyers may feel freed from the strictures of self, family, and society, discovering new and seemingly heretical truths. It can be tempting to join them, blithely throwing aside the conventions of our role as therapists.

The field of psychedelic therapy and research has known its share of scandals. It's easy to blame outside forces for the stigma around psychedelics: the sensationalism of the media, or the scaremongering tactics of government agencies. Boundary crossing and ethical violations have been rife in this field from the beginning, however, and have influenced public perception.

This is by no means unique to psychedelic therapy. Because the therapist in these sessions has an inordinate amount of power, though, damaging behavior can occur more easily—and be more destructive when it occurs. The boundary violations of therapists and guides have wounded many. At the same time, they have denigrated the profession itself. Psychedelics are now associated in the public imagination with cult dynamics and sexual abuse.

Some of the therapists or researchers in question might be unrepentant narcissists. Sometimes, though, we see a fellow guide publicly reckoning with a past misdeed. In these cases, the clinician usually describes themselves acting against their own better judgment. These tales are instructive, as even the most experienced guides can lose their way.

This generally relates to Jung's (1951/1968) idea of the *shadow*, the disowned parts of the self. All of us feel shame—at least those of us who are psychologically healthy—but this emotion is difficult to tolerate. Over time, we repress the shameful facets of ourselves. In twilight they lurk, operating below the threshold of awareness to influence our thinking and behavior. Good-hearted people can find themselves acting out in ways antithetical to their most deeply held values.

APPLYING ETHICS TO PSYCHEDELIC-ASSISTED THERAPY

Many themes related to ethical practice are already covered in therapeutic codes. However, there are specific considerations for implementing these into psychedelic therapy. In the current climate, psychedelic-assisted therapy may exist in a quasi-legal or *underground* context. This ambiguity does not suggest that it's permissible to cut corners regarding client care.

Consent and Confidentiality

Informed consent is standard. Most professionals are required to give patients or clients a form to sign, detailing the practitioner's obligations and the client's recourse to reporting complaints if they don't live up to this standard. Psychedelic work, given that it initiates people into entirely new phenomenological states, necessitates a higher standard of informed consent. Prospective clients need thorough preparation, and should be offered a menu of possibilities for their experience (including possible adverse events). The client needs to consent to these risks, as well as agree to any special needs the therapist has (such as remaining anonymous, for example). Practitioners can limit their liability by getting a signed and dated informed consent form, or a packet of forms, that covers all of these risks.

Many professions legislate the need for client confidentiality. Neither the client's identity nor what they share should be discussed outside of the therapeutic relationship. Professionals are required to be discreet. Obviously, this requirement is intensified when working with drugs that have social stigma. It could have legal ramifications if clients were to become exposed, or could create reputational damage.

Certain professionals are *mandatory reporters*, though. Laws in the United States require a psychotherapist to contact authorities if a client presents a danger to themselves, to others, and/or if the therapist suspects that a known child is being abused. If a client tells their psychotherapist the full name and location of someone who abused them in childhood, for instance, and if that abuser currently has access to children, the therapist is required to report this. Similarly, suicidal or violent tendencies can be discussed and worked with in therapy, but if the client has the means—and a plan—the therapist needs to consider reporting this to authorities. In psychedelic experiences, clients may freely discuss traumas and other issues. However, mandatory reporting requirements still hold. This issue must be discussed in advance and covered by written acknowledgement or consent, and reminders can be delivered at the appropriate time.

Romantic and Sexual Boundaries

Romantic or sexual relationships between therapist and client are always off-limits. This commonplace prohibition is one of the most commonly transgressed, and the psychedelic therapy world is no exception. In fact, altered states of consciousness may invite boundary confusion, and cause seemingly irresistible primal energies to arise. The sense of having accessed deeper or more profound truths may incline us to throw aside boundaries, making both client and therapist temporarily *antinomian*—rejecting socially established morality. Clients may disinhibit in their journey, and this is healthy and necessary, but the therapist shouldn't join them there. Our job is to hold space.

The therapist, committed to not acting out sexual desires with clients, can nonetheless help the client to befriend the primordial force of sexuality. Exploring the body in psychedelic states may mean discovering sensations in the genitals, an awakening of sexual desire, and other such hungers for contact and intimacy that are often socially stigmatized. A client may want to disrobe, or describe a newly dawning sense of attraction toward the therapist. The therapist's job at this point is to normalize these responses, to be unoffended, and to remind the client of preexisting agreements and boundaries. It's to be celebrated that they're connecting with the disowned parts of themselves and awakening their vitality. Shaking off the shame associated with sexuality can be an outcome of effective psychedelic therapy. A solid boundary between therapist and client makes these explorations safe and productive.

One thorny question in this area relates to romantic relationships after the therapeutic relationship is over. The rules around these situations vary. The American Psychological Association (2017), for instance, states in its *Ethical Principles of Psychologists and Code of Conduct* that psychologists should not have a sexual relationship with a former client, unless at least 2 years have elapsed since services were terminated. This should only occur, though, "in the most unusual circumstances" (Standard 10.08). The American Association for Marriage and Family Therapy (2015) states flatly, "Sexual intimacy with former clients . . . is prohibited" (Standard 1.5). The OHA, overseeing legal psilocybin-assisted therapy in Oregon, says,

> No romantic relationships, sexual contact, or sexual intimacy with clients is permitted during any stage of psilocybin services including preparatory, administration, and integration sessions. In addition, sexual contact or romantic relationships with clients, or their partners or immediate family members, is prohibited for one year after the facilitator–client relationship has been formally terminated. (Oregon Health Authority, 2024a)

Clearly this is an area that requires intention and care, particularly as psychedelic work can increase the potential for *erotic transference*—the tendency for clients to develop a physical attraction toward their therapist. The journeyer's safety and personal growth needs to be prioritized above all else.

Multiple Relationships

Another situation relevant to many therapeutic endeavors is *multiple relationships*, when therapists treat someone they know from elsewhere. It's generally thought that clients benefit from anonymity. In the presence of someone known to us, we may—consciously or unconsciously—hold back aspects of our process. For instance, if the therapist is a friend, or someone we know from church, we might be reticent to tell them our full history. We may not be transparent in regard to our emotions, especially how we feel about people the therapist also knows. If the journeyer knows they're going to see this person in another setting—say, at a dance party, or a 12-step meeting—it could be more challenging to be fully open and vulnerable. This can impinge on a direct engagement with one's inner life, which is necessary for healing.

However, there are those who distrust the aforementioned approach. The notion that helpers should be unknowable professionals outside the client's social sphere is a modern invention. Some clients report that working with someone who understands them, with whom they share cultural referents, is healing. For some, it may be important that the healer *isn't* a stranger, as this can redress the power imbalances inherent in the therapy relationship.

Another consideration relates to alternative therapies, like somatic approaches. These modalities often first develop in fringe communities of people. Finding a provider we don't already know may not be feasible, especially if we don't live in a large urban center. Practitioners might find it necessary to ethically negotiate multiple relationships.

All of these factors are even more relevant when it comes to psychedelic-assisted therapy. These medicines foster disinhibition, and clients may say or do things they later find embarrassing. On MDMA, for instance, a person may have little interest in self-editing; on psilocybin, they may not have a choice. Journeyers may feel unmasked, sharing pieces of their history or circumstances of their current life they later wish they could take back.

Our perspective is that multiple relationships aren't to be avoided per se but approached with intention and clarity. Complications can certainly arise. Again, the goal should always be protecting the client's experience, first and foremost. When I've [Joshua] worked with people in my community, I always name our multiple roles, and ask the client how they feel about this. I've developed a shtick where I talk about wearing "multiple hats," pantomiming taking off the *friend* or *colleague* hat and putting on the *therapist* one. I make it clear that my only goal in this role is supporting and protecting them. Reminding them about confidentiality is also important here. At the end of our time, I make it clear we will exit the roles of therapist and client as the session concludes.

However, it is especially challenging for clients to be themselves if the therapist is also their teacher, their employer, or in any role that has *evaluative authority* over them. The client may withhold things if being fully open could compromise their opportunities for advancement, or make them look "crazy" in the eyes of someone they need to impress. In fact, the OHA's (2022) *Ethical Principles* state unequivocally: "Facilitators should not provide services to people over whom they have supervisory, evaluative, or other authority" (Section 7).

We should also use caution if a potential client is a partner, friend, or a relation of another client. People who benefit from working with us may be excited to refer others to our practice. In these situations, I always ask, "Is there any way in which this could potentially affect our therapy?" I remind the client that this other person may end up talking about them, and I could potentially hear unflattering things about them. Some clients feel fine about this, and insist it will not jeopardize their unconditional trust in our relationship. In psychedelic-assisted work this is especially important. A healing journey can feel *liberating*, and it's not uncommon to hear journeyers say, "I wish so-and-so could have this experience too." It could be tempting for a client to start referring everyone they know. We should coach them to consider the potential ramifications. And we can always refer this new person to another provider.

Power Differentials

All therapies involve power differentials. In the psychedelic experience, with its characteristic vulnerability and regression, these are intensified. Any therapeutic relationship represents a difference in role power, with the therapist often imagined as an all-knowing expert and the client a passive recipient of their interventions. There are various ways to undermine this—and undermining it is an important part of effective therapy—but there will still be an inherent inequality in these roles. The power imbalance can reactivate developmental wounding for the client, increasing their dependency on the therapist. While this does present possible avenues for corrective experiences, it can easily become disenfranchising for the client.

It's important to note that having greater power in a relationship isn't necessarily bad. If we use this power for good, it may be a wise investment on the part of the journeyer. In fact, power is often poorly understood in the hierarchical societies of the modern West. We have maxims like Lord Acton's "Power tends to corrupt, and absolute power corrupts absolutely" (Creighton, 1906,

p. 372). Examples abound of people drunk on status and influence doing horrible things. Yet it may be truer to say that power doesn't necessarily corrupt but it always *reveals*. In other words, one's unaddressed shadow will emerge when one attains role power. We should carefully examine ourselves and our motives as we gain power (Barstow, 2015).

Being powerful needn't make others powerless. Starhawk (1989) describes healthy empowerment as *power from within*, emphasizing that this is crucial for living fully. She also makes a distinction between *power over* versus *power with*. Fully manifesting one's life force doesn't require disempowering others. Power is often misconstrued as the domination of others, but it can just as easily uplift others. Being in our own power in healthy, egalitarian ways can invite others to be powerful too.

All of these considerations require intention and ethical discernment. It can be easy to lapse into a *laissez-faire* approach, especially if a mystical naivete makes us want to simply "trust the process." Two crucial determinants of positive outcomes in journeys are *set* and *setting*: set is the psychological state of the person taking the psychedelic, while setting signifies the environment in which the journey takes place. We believe that ethical constructs are necessary boundaries that help create an optimal container, affecting the client's trust in the process (set) as well as the environment they are in (setting—which includes us, of course).

ETHICAL CONSIDERATIONS FOR SYSTEMIC INEQUALITY

One must also consider the power that one is accorded in society, sometimes arbitrarily. Systemic inequalities proliferate through the modern world, and these can determine material outcomes and impact psychological health. In the United States, discrimination based on race, class, gender, and other factors limits one's prospects in life. Historically, certain people faced subjugation, humiliation, and bodily harm from the dominant group, solely due to immutable characteristics. This legacy of oppression gave rise to enduring cultural norms that continue to punish people for being born too dark, too poor, the wrong gender, or being attracted to the wrong sex.

The distorted prism of stereotypes, which objectifies people in ways both denigrating and complimentary, makes it difficult to discover a sense of belonging. Being a target of harassment and violence hinders the development of a sense of safety. The experience of marginalization may constrain one's *self-efficacy*—the sense that one can effectively act, accomplish goals, and better one's life circumstances (sometimes referred to as a sense of *agency*). Oppression can also create an *external locus of control*, where we perceive our fate as being in the hands of others (this is differentiated from an *internal locus of control*, where we feel like the captain of our own ship). Mental health is associated with a sense of self-efficacy (Bandura, 1982) and an internal locus of control (Rotter, 1966). When things feel out of our control, something in us falters.

The debilitating effects of persecution affect people in many different identity categories, even for those who may benefit from systemic inequality in other ways. Living in a world rife with separation and discord harms each and every one of us. Nobody asked for things to be this way. No one chose to be born into a world that systematically privileges some and immiserates others for things entirely outside of their control. This recognition can be liberating for those we serve—as well as for ourselves. It's possible, even likely, that cultural or historical trauma will emerge in psychedelic work. As guides, we must be prepared to navigate this.

Journeyers might dredge up intergenerational trauma, wounding passed down through genetic and cultural imprints. Research has shown that the children of Holocaust survivors have a physiological response to stress that differs from the general population, despite never being exposed to the horrific traumas of their parents (Yehuda & Lehrner, 2018). Studies on mice, which have a similar nervous system to our own, have found evidence for the transgenerational transmission of *triggers*—somatosensory cues that initiate a fear response—five generations down the line (Dias & Ressler, 2013). Each client may be carrying a unique legacy of ancestral wounding.

Marginalized groups have historically suffered abuse and mistreatment in the medical system. Black Americans were subjected to unethical medical experimentation, such as the infamous Tuskegee experiment. Along with Indigenous people (and others), they experience significant health disparities compared to White people (Institute of Medicine, 2002). Racial minorities have been targeted by forced sterilization campaigns. So have the mentally ill. The model for mental illness itself was rife with gender bias in the early days of psychiatry. The term "hysteria" refers to the womb (from the Greek, *hyster*); the increased prevalence of mental illness in women was thought to stem from a malfunctioning uterus. The dominant culture has tended to see ethnic minorities, sexual minorities, women, and the underclass as somehow deviant or defective, and in need of fixing.

Even psychedelic therapy has championed bias and stigmatization. Grof's *LSD Psychotherapy* (1980), an otherwise worthwhile primer on psychedelic therapy protocols, features a section where the author posits that psychedelics could be useful in treating the "deviation" of homosexuality (p. 244). This kind of psychedelic conversion therapy should horrify us. Healers can unwittingly become agents of a sick society, maltreating vulnerable people. It is to be expected that clients may mistrust us, and our efforts. We must ensure that our field reflects ethical values.

Working Across Difference

At times we *work across difference*, when the therapist's social location doesn't match that of their client. The two may differ in terms of race, gender, class, or other identity characteristics, and it can be important to speak to this early in the relationship. Some clients have powerful corrective experiences working with someone who differs from them, but who is unconditionally caring and supportive. Other clients may realize they need a therapist who shares their race, sexuality, gender identity, religion, or class background, someone who *gets* them and intuitively understands this aspect of their life. In either case, it won't be helpful to consider this an abstract political concern, or busily defend against guilt or shame around our own identities.

The participants in psychedelic research are overwhelmingly White, middle to upper class, and include few immigrants, transgendered people, or other minorities. Because of this skewed representation, we simply don't know how generalizable the findings are, and shouldn't assume that all journeyers will benefit—or benefit to the same degree—as these studies suggest.

Although we want the greatest number of people possible to benefit, psychedelic-assisted therapy is an uneconomical treatment model. It requires many, many hours of professional labor, making it prohibitively expensive for the majority of people. Hopefully, increasing acceptance of these treatments will force insurers to cover them (this is part of why empirical validation is so important). Many providers choose to offer sliding scale, reduced-fee, or pro bono slots to some percentage of clients. The OHA requires Oregonians offering psilocybin services to develop an "equity plan," a system each practitioner creates for their practice to serve a diverse population (Oregon Health Authority, 2024b). Something akin to this could be important for all psychedelic guides to create.

EXPERIENTIAL ETHICS AND PSYCHEDELIC-ASSISTED THERAPY

Psychedelic journeys explore terra incognita, and the guide must have some direct knowledge of how to explore. It's generally thought that we shouldn't guide what we don't know. If a therapist is unfamiliar with a particular psychedelic agent, they should consider the ethics of holding space for a journey with that medicine. Many psychedelic therapy trainings don't feature an experiential component, either because it's illegal or because it's elective. We hope this changes in the coming years, making this section of the chapter obsolete. In the meantime, aspiring psychedelic therapists need to weigh the ethics of extralegal drug experimentation, on the one hand, and guiding journeys they may not fully grasp, on the other. A therapist who has personal experience with psychedelics will know that a client may struggle mightily before breaking through. The therapist's lived experience conveys a great deal to the journeyer, steadying and stabilizing them.

An experienced therapist is also less likely to judge the journey, knowing that things may be fast or slow, loud or quiet, cerebral or emotional—and will oscillate between these polarities throughout. We are not guiding in the sense of leading someone to a preordained destination. We are qualified as guides because we understand something of the terrain. We may not have traversed this particular landscape before; and yet, we are familiar with the general weather patterns, the peaks and valleys, the watercourses, and how to thrive in the wild. We help the client access the inner resources needed to make the journey.

Some approaches involve the guide taking medicine alongside the journeyer. Legitimate mentorship lineages exist in this style of practice, but these practitioners generally have *long* experiential training behind them. We don't recommend this for new guides, or for people without training in this specific style. The steadying influence of the guide can be harder to access when both parties are inebriated.

We have to respect the client's beliefs, the unique way their embodied psyche frames the imagery, emotion, and sensation in order to create new meaning. We must trust that their inner resources—in a sense, other guides—will emerge to hold them. Part of our ethical commitment is to avoid becoming their guru, referring them back to their own innate strength and resilience while in an expanded state.

At times we may watch our clients circuitously swirl around an obvious insight, or become lost in a maze of associations. We may be tempted to offer an interpretation to resolve the tension. But these gaps in understanding are seedbeds for their own emerging truth, and we should avoid trying to fill in the blanks. While sometimes it may be necessary to rescue them, the accomplished guide often does *less*, having patience with the process as it stochastically moves toward unforeseen ends.

The client's spirituality is important here. The medical model of psychedelic therapy is in danger of omitting the sacred, even though research has repeatedly shown that a *mystical-type experience* is associated with more substantive and enduring change (Griffiths et al., 2008). We need to safeguard this pathway for healing and transformation. Each individual has a *higher power*—something greater than the self—whether it be nature, a God or gods, ancestors, or a principle of intelligent unfolding in the universe or cosmos (such as evolution). Connecting with this power is often central to the psychedelic experience, as guides discover in their own personal journeys. A myopic focus on biological or biographical aspects can harm not just the journeyer's experience but also psychedelic therapy as a field.

OVERSIGHT FOR PSYCHEDELIC THERAPISTS

We shouldn't do this work alone. The presence of a second therapist can be a boon for psychedelic work, for both practitioner(s) and client. Having another competent professional in the journey space not only provides the client with additional support, it also gives the therapist an extra set of hands, a chance to "tag out" after intense moments in the journey, and a colleague to debrief with afterward. The second therapist is also a source of oversight preventing ethical transgressions, protecting the client while keeping both practitioners honest. Most studies demonstrating clinical efficacy for psychedelics involve therapist teams, and this arrangement may be the ideal one for psychedelic work.

However, the cost of therapist teams may be prohibitive, and for other reasons this may not be realistic. Another way to avoid doing the work alone, then, is through supervision, mentorship, and consultation. As mentioned, expanded states can invite boundary confusion, relational intensity, and other dynamics that pose challenges to one's ethics. Having someone to check in with—a trusted person to hear all the gritty details of the session—is invaluable.

Shamanic training in many indigenous contexts entails years or decades of mentorship, a thoroughgoing initiation into guiding plant medicine experiences. Such cultures have developed frameworks for working with expanded states over centuries of experimentation and refinement. In the modern West, we have none of this cultural context, and few elders to accurately assess a practitioner's readiness. Months-long training programs—particularly those without an experiential component—cannot redress this deficiency. Psychedelic therapists need mentors, people who have negotiated the ethical quandaries that arise. We need colleagues and peers to recount experiences with, paying attention to emerging issues and receiving support to handle them responsibly.

Sometimes we hear about ethical misdeeds committed by other providers. If we learn this information from a client, confidentiality is the first consideration. We shouldn't come forward with it unless the client gives explicit permission in the form of a signed release. If we hear about it "through the grapevine," we should carefully consider how to respond. This is another area where one's licensure may proscribe a particular response. If we hear about a violation of the codes governing marriage and family therapy committed by a fellow licensed marriage and family therapist (LMFT), for instance, we are legally obligated to report it to our board. Reporting to a board or publicly commenting on ethical transgressions in other instances is something that should be carefully considered, as it can entail inestimable professional and reputational damage. Of course, the priority is the client's well-being, at any cost—this one as well as future clients seeking ethically sound treatment.

In psychedelic-assisted therapy, there's no licensing board to report to. Therefore, community accountability is an important principle. We can consider approaching the individual directly, communicating our concern. We can also invite other colleagues into a dialogue, using the rupture to strengthen a collective commitment to ethical practice.

CONCLUSION

Ethics is a preeminent concern for all helping professions but especially for psychedelic-assisted therapy. Recent scandals illuminate the need for this to be central to our understanding of these drugs and their uses. If we respect these medicines, and the potential for healing and transformation they represent, we must do everything in our power to create a strong container for the work. We must compassionately interrogate our motives, remaining vigilant and steadfast as we keep to our commitments. We must make sure the journeyer comes first, protecting them from our shadow as we introduce them to their inner healer.

CHAPTER 3

The Body in Psychedelic Therapy

After they begin to wake up, they learn to trust their own sensations. One can learn not to restrict one's view; to feel oneself as a member of this planet we all live on.
—CHARLOTTE SELVER

Connection with the body is fundamental to our sense of self. We establish this connection early in life through the loving touch of caregivers. As we mature, the support of our family, our community, and the protective environment of our culture and institutions allow us to inhabit our bodies healthily. If any of these structures should falter, however, we can become alienated from an embodied sense of who we are.

The body is a relational organism. The nonverbal realm of touch, sensation, and movement shows us our place in the family of things. Bodies are communicating all the time. We implicitly read people's micro-expressions and posture, telling us without words how we are being received. We see in the body language of others whether we are welcomed. Our bodies broadcast the hurts and rejections of the past. Whether we know it or not, we live a somatic life.

Somatic comes from *soma* (σῶμα), the word for "body" in Ancient Greek. We understand soma to encompass the physical, emotional, mental, and spiritual aspects of being, for all the layers of human experience are fundamentally embodied and integrated. Soma is a highly intelligent resource.

Somatic psychology centers on bodily experience—physical sensations, emotions, autonomic responses, patterns of tension or holding, and so on—as an integral aspect of our cognitive life. Unconscious behaviors can be brought into awareness through somatic practices involving movement, breath, and mindfulness, fostering a conscious connection between mind and body.

As somatic therapists, we help our clients learn the language of the body, with its immense vocabulary of tension patterns, subtle movements, and sensations. This process takes time and patience, but in a therapeutic environment, clients can learn this language and uncover the stories hidden beneath the surface.

SOMATIC MARKERS

The neuroscientist Antonio Damasio (2005) hypothesized that emotion influences decision making via physiological responses, such as the rapid heart rate often associated with anxiety. He called these bodily cues *somatic markers*. According to Damasio, every time we decide or make choices we do so emotionally and somatically. The body "marks options and outcomes with a positive or negative signal that narrows the decision-making space and increases the probability that the action will conform to past experience" (Damasio, 2003, p. 148). Somatic markers can include changes in heart rhythm, skin conductance, muscle tone, perspiration, and other nervous system shifts. Over time, we associate our somatic markers with specific situations and their past outcomes, which influence our subsequent decisions.

Identifying and understanding our own somatic markers can powerfully contribute to our self-knowledge and the therapeutic change process. The body has a primary role in shaping our responses to the world, and learning how to listen to the body is vitally important to our growth.

Most of us are not taught to listen to our bodies. Western culture, in particular, tends to dismiss the body's signals. We are taught to override tiredness or hunger, ignore pain, numb ourselves to sensations, and tune out sensory perceptions. A rich world of inner experience is always humming in the background of consciousness if we would only notice it. Many of us learn that our bodily experience is out of control, dangerous, untrustworthy, or will lead us astray. So, we exert top-down control, sorting our feelings and sensations into familiar categories that align with our limited conceptual frameworks. As a result, the body's language often remains inscrutable to the conscious mind. And so, we live our lives without the body's wisdom.

Somatic therapy, however, reveals that body, mind, and spirit are interconnected. The self is not a ghost in the machine of the body. We do not *have* a body; we *are* a body. We think, feel, sense, and move through the world as one being, yet we perceive ourselves as an amalgam of isolated parts. But our lived experience leaves somatic markers, hovering just below the level of conscious awareness, awaiting our notice. A particular scent can suddenly trigger a rush of memory with associated sensations, emotions, and sense perceptions.

A vivid example of a somatic marker comes to mind: the scent of my [Manuela] grandmother instantly evokes a deep, complex memory. When I catch a whiff of her perfume—a sweet, heavy fragrance called Opium—I feel her presence enveloping me. I sense her love and miss her profoundly. I recall the crackly sound of her smoky voice, her delicate fingers stroking my hair, and the warmth and safety radiating from her gaze. My awareness settles gently in my belly. Tears well up as I remember her grief and resilience as a survivor of World War II and her steely resolve to endure. Our connection stretches back through time, linking me to my mother and my great-grandmother—a lineage of women carrying the weight of accumulated trauma. The devastating impact of the Weimar Republic, the Nazi regime, the Holocaust, and postwar Germany all flow through me, burning in my stomach, tightening my jaw, and my tears fall. The longing to feel her touch on my hair evokes comfort and pain—the complex history of my family's somatic memory. It is alive within me. It lives in my body.

Somatic markers are living memories, intricate paths woven through us. They can reflect ancestral knowledge, heavy with the weight of history. These intergenerational marks connect us to the emotions and experiences of those who came before us, shaping our understanding of self and identity. Each marker carries the echoes of past struggles and triumphs, inviting us to honor the legacy of resilience that flows through our soma. In this way, they act as a bridge, linking our present experiences to the rich tapestry of our lineage, reminding us of the strength and depth that reside within.

Understanding our somatic markers can reveal how emotions and bodily sensations influence our decision making. Past emotional experiences, regardless of their nature, inform our present choices. By exploring these markers, we integrate our sense of self and recognize how we've been shaped from the inside out. For instance, the anxious flutter of butterflies before going on stage carries a different significance than the anticipation felt while waiting for a loved one. Similarly, the warmth of someone's touch can evoke memories of a cherished embrace, while a song from childhood may bring back long-buried feelings of joy or sadness.

Emotions, images, beliefs, hopes, and fears are not just abstract cognition. They are encoded in the body. By approaching common physical side effects of psychedelic intoxication as potential somatic markers, therapists can dive deeply into the core issues showing up in the body's reactions. Nausea may be an opening into the client's disgust at themselves or others. Vomiting can be a chance to purge a habitual pattern that is no longer serving them. Or *involuntary movements*—the body moving on its own, like in trembling or jerking—may be incomplete self-protective actions that we can support to complete.

In psychedelic therapy, we experience these powerful markers with enhanced *interoception*, the awareness of internal bodily sensations. We access vivid sensory stimuli, and deep inner knowing. Somatic phenomena—manifesting in the luminous and evocative space of expanded states—can give us powerful insight into how the past has shaped us, as well as how the past continues to shape our future. Without incorporating this bodily knowledge, we can't fully heal.

Try This: Identifying Somatic Markers

Reflecting on your somatic markers can give you a greater sense of how to guide others into becoming more sensitive. Reflect for a moment on this:

- Think of an unpleasant person or situation from your early life. It doesn't have to be the worst trauma you ever suffered or the person who hurt you the most, just something or someone that created a negative feeling in the past.
- What life decisions did you make in response to this? What did you avoid because of it?
- Think about these decisions. Now, put your attention on your body.
- Can you feel the effects of these choices right now in your

body? What do they feel like? Tightness? Heat? Pressure? Where can you feel them?
- Which somatic markers from your past do you recognize?
- Do you notice a link from the past experience to your current life?

When I reflect on my path as a therapist, I see how the suffering of my family, the legacy of fascism, and my bicultural identity all led me to examine the embodied responses that shaped my beliefs. This placed me on a path to help others.

In psychedelic-assisted therapy, the client opens into a depth of experience that touches their somatic markers—and can also trigger yours. These moments are important to recognize. They are subtle, energetic shifts that can impact your guiding abilities.

Expanded states also provide opportunities to *change* somatic markers. In the preparation phase, we encourage clients to investigate their bodies, giving them a deeper understanding of these somatic markers' origin and associated beliefs. In the dosing session, more adaptive bodily impressions may be formed. In the integration phase, we explore these shifts in embodiment and determine how they will bring about lasting therapeutic change. As the body changes, we change.

THE FELT SENSE

Our family, culture, and society influence our beliefs and perceptions. We show who we are through gestures, posture, tone of voice, rhythm of speech, gait, and so on. We express or withhold our emotions, perhaps even to ourselves. Learning to read the soma—our own body and the bodies of others—is like learning a new language. The nonverbal style of our embodied experience is unintelligible when we are not taught to listen to it.

In his seminal book *Focusing*, Eugene Gendlin (1981) called this language the *felt sense*. The felt sense is beyond any emotion or body sensation. It is a deeper knowing of one's bodily wisdom, a way of sensing the totality of experience in an integrated gestalt of sensation, emotion, words, and images. A particular phrase from the therapist may elicit a sudden feeling of sadness in the client, then a mental image of someone from their past who used the same phrase, an associated ache in the chest, heaviness in the limbs, the realization that they miss this person, a sharpness of breath that gives them a sense they could cry. This organically unfolding mandala of inner experience is the felt sense.

The psychedelic therapist must be fluent in the language of the body. To attain this, we cultivate a set of highly attuned observational skills, as well as traverse our own inner landscape. We can't help a client access their soma unless we can access our own. Because bodily states are nonverbal, psychedelic therapists must be trained to read even the subtlest somatic cues. The training ground is our experiential exploration of the felt sense.

Try This: The Soma as Is

- Take a moment to let yourself slow down and turn your attention inward.
- Now, without overly controlling it, allow your breath to become soft.
- With no goal or agenda, arrive in your soma *as it is* right now.
- Invite your body to be fully present. What do you notice?
- Linger and stay inward for another moment. Sustain your attention.
- Can you stay with your soma *as it is*, with no attempt to change anything?

- What arises as you do so?
- Allow your attention to turn outward again. What differences can you perceive?

SOMATICS AND PSYCHEDELICS

When we think of psychedelic journeys, often what comes to mind are kaleidoscopic visions, cosmic insights, and cathartic emotional releases. But beneath these wildly explosive displays lies another realm, ancient as the earth and wise as nature itself: the body. Psychedelics open our perceptual fields in ways that conventional psychotherapy cannot. They allow us to sink below the surface of ordinary awareness, unearthing what has been buried, disavowed, or hidden. This enables healing. The biochemical changes that psychedelics elicit may unlock a deeper somatic awareness, newfound perceptions, and a depth of feeling in the body.

Classical psychedelics (such as psilocybin, LSD, and mescaline) primarily bind to serotonin receptors, particularly the 5-HT2A receptor, influencing our perception of somatosensory states. We may experience a strange sense of lightness or heaviness, changes in muscle tone, tension in our jaw, nausea, or distortions to *proprioception*: our awareness of the body's position in space. The cumulative effect of such perceptual changes is often referred to in psychedelic work as a "body load."

Many people regard this powerfully physical aspect of the psychedelic experience as a mere side effect, but it can invite the journeyer into a deeper connection with the body. As one client said, "My body is safe for the first time." Previous to this, she had been unable to access an embodied experience of safety, no matter how much cognitive understanding she gained from conventional psychotherapy. But on psychedelics, her familiar protective mechanisms of avoidance and cognitive compartmentalization finally let go and allowed for a deep union with her body. Safety was no longer an idea or a yearning but an embodied reality she could feel. Only a new *experience* could affect such a change.

Case Study: Tabor

Psychedelics melt the perceived boundary between mind and body, eliciting vulnerable and tender emotional states and a new intimacy with oneself. Another of my [Manuela] clients, Tabor, was able to access a sense of aliveness and sensuality in their body, one they had not experienced prior to the psychedelic journey.

When I met with Tabor, embodiment was a foreign idea to them. Tabor's abuse as a preteen, and shame about their sexuality, had a devastating impact. This shame led to self-harming behavior and a general rejection of their body. Tabor experienced crushing depression and extreme anxiety whenever they were in an intimate relationship. Embodiment was a foreign idea. Their body had become a place of disgust, confinement, and torment. Even in somatic therapy, Tabor struggled to be in their body. Most physical experiences were met with vigilance and memories of abuse.

In the psychedelic session, they were finally able to relax and discover their soma. The novel somatosensory awareness of the psychedelic state shifted these deeply entrenched patterns, allowing Tabor to feel at home in their own skin. In the integration phase, this experience became a new reference point from which Tabor could now be in their body without memories of trauma arising.

For clients who have become disembodied due to sexual trauma or early attachment wounds, this newfound connection with the body can feel like coming home. Emotional barriers and compensatory patterns can be *felt* rather than understood. A sensorial aliveness and interoceptive clarity come online, inviting the client to trust the knowledge of the body. States of deep relaxation, acceptance of feelings, and new capacities for sensation often result.

Case Study: Annie

Annie was another client who'd become alienated from her soma. "I hate feeling my body," she'd often say, using words like "yucky," "bad," "uncomfortable," and "repulsive" when attempting to work with body sensations. She loathed mindfulness practices. Her mind would wander, her attention restless. Exercising in the gym, a strict and repetitive regimen, was the only form of body awareness she could tolerate. A high-functioning executive, Annie liked order and routine and could provide very well for herself. She'd come from a stable family in a middle-class neighborhood. But she had never found a long-term relationship, or started a family of her own, as she'd secretly longed for.

Annie came into therapy with a dreary and heavy sense that life was moving by without her. She was depressed when not working and had, in recent months, become anxious about her presentations at work. These fits of worry became full-blown anxiety attacks, where she would black out for the entire presentation and find herself alone in the bathroom, shaking and throwing up.

In our intake session, Annie disclosed sexual boundary violations with a family friend when she was a small child, and again from a boyfriend later in life—but dismissed their significance. "It was all OK," she said with a little smile. Our work together focused on fostering awareness of body sensations and her tendency to push them away. Even though Annie did not like the somatic work, she appreciated the insight she gained into her coping mechanisms. She became increasingly curious about why she was so averse to her own body.

In her first ketamine session, Annie discovered a sense of ease and release in her body, a lightness and sensuality she had never known. Her accustomed resistance to sensation melted away, and she was moved to tears for missing this beautiful experience of her own body.

In later stages of the journey, she confronted old memories of shame as an adolescent, revisiting the inappropriate advances and sexual violations of male relatives. Pain and discomfort arose as she remembered withdrawing from the unwanted touch, the confusion around feeling both pleasure and terror at once. Her body contracted and contorted as if she were pushing the invasive men away, moving through the somatic markers of the abuse.

Noticing her discomfort, I encouraged her to follow the movements. "Trust your body right now. Just take it one movement at a time."

Annie's clenched hand slowly opened, and a deep growl emerged from her throat. Then she began to sob. Layers of grief washed through her. She was letting go, allowing the deeply held fear and resistance to fall away. Her hands trembled, then her knees, until finally her arms and legs were all shaking.

"Stay with your body," I said. "Just follow what's here."

Annie's hand flew out, reaching for me.

I drew a long, slow breath and took her hand.

I responded to her reach for comfort, gently encouraging her with somatic directives to fully engage with her experience.

Stabilized by the contact, Annie's sobbing ebbed away, her chest rising and falling in a flowing, wavelike pattern. Her pain was abating.

I mirrored her fluid breathing as her body continued to settle. Then, a deeper, more spontaneous breath appeared, a tender, wavelike breath, and I knew she had arrived back in her body.

Annie opened her eyes, and there was light in them. Tears streamed down her face.

I crossed her arms over her chest, letting her hold herself.

She lay there, smiling, in a state of inseparable union with her body, traversing an inner landscape she had never explored. The innate intelligence of her soma had awakened.

In our integration sessions, Annie became deeply engaged with the somatic therapy process. A whole new appreciation for embodied existence had emerged. She began to explore yoga and dance, practices of somatic enjoyment. The ketamine session opened her to the possibility of experiencing sensation, without the fear and resistance that had long entrapped her.

Annie came to fully embrace herself, recognizing her wholeness amid the wounding she'd suffered. Over time, she was able to approach traumatic memories with curiosity and self-compassion, recognizing her resistance as a protective barrier. The journey had enabled a profound shift, leading to a deep connection with her somatic intelligence.

"TRUST THE PROCESS" MEANS TRUSTING THE SOMA

In psychedelic-assisted therapy, somatic and emotional responses can be deeply intertwined. The healing impact of psychedelic experiences often occurs bottom-up, outside of our cognitive understanding, and below the level of conscious awareness. To fully benefit from this work, we must relinquish our need for control and our agenda for a particular outcome. "Trust the process" is axiomatic within psychedelic therapy circles, but how is this accomplished? What exactly are we putting our trust in?

To trust the process requires that we trust the soma. The inner healing intelligence includes the intelligence of the body. Teaching clients to trust their soma becomes the basis for opening to the intensity of expanded states. When we can rely on our embodied being, we peel back the obfuscating mask of ego, revealing the insidious patterns of tension, the hidden impacts of trauma, and the latent capacities for resilience. In other words, we see what is happening beneath the surface. In trusting the soma, clients learn to befriend their entire being, even those aspects tethered to pain and avoidance. Clients often report experiences of their body dissolving and then being made anew, recast in a form more aligned to their true nature.

If this sense of trust is revisited in the integration phase, and stabilized through body-centered practices like yoga or somatic therapy, the client may be able to preserve their new level of embodiment in a lasting way. This trust in the soma can be accessed in the integration phase through inquiries from the therapist: "Can you remember that unconditional sense of trust you felt in your journey? As you think about that, what do you notice in your body now?" The somatic markers associated with this trust can be used as reference points in daily life, somatosensory reminders of insights from the journey that transcend thought and language.

We tend to control our experience even in therapy. We talk *about* a problem, seeking pragmatic solutions and instant outcomes. We can become impatient with life. Our accustomed mental habits have established neural networks that reinforce habitual behaviors. But when we have space and time to sink into our experience, we can connect with the organic process of life unfolding. Both somatic psychotherapy and psychedelic-assisted therapy emphasize the slow, deliberate observation of our total experience. This is how we access the inner healing intelligence.

DECRYPTING THE BODY'S MESSAGES IN THE PSYCHEDELIC EXPERIENCE

Psychedelics reveal and amplify somatic markers—the physical signals that accompany our emotional responses. These can manifest in myriad ways: changes in breathing patterns, temperature fluctuations, muscular tension, and so on. For the uninitiated, these phenomena might appear to be mere drug side effects, but for the somatically attuned therapist, they are gateways to the client's emotional and psychological landscape.

Imagine a session where the client reports a sudden flush of heat through their chest. It could be tempting to dismiss this as the drug impacting their circulatory system, but to a somatically aware therapist it may in fact indicate an emotional release or a discharge of pent-up energy—a breakthrough moment. We can bring about deep and lasting change by tracking these somatic markers in the client's conscious awareness.

Documenting somatic markers provides a map for the terrain of the journey. We can write them down as they appear and then analyze and reflect upon them in the integration phase. This enriches the therapeutic process and enhances the safety and comfort of the client, who will likely feel seen and heard on a visceral level, perhaps for the first time. Examining such somatosensory phenomena in the daylight of ordinary consciousness may help us decode and interpret these messages, which are often cryptic when they first appear.

CONCLUSION

In the field of psychedelic-assisted therapy, a vital aspect of the work is gradually being recognized—the language of the body during these profound journeys of the mind. It is commonplace for clients to experience aches, flushes, chills, or involuntary movement as they traverse challenging emotional territories. By acknowledging and supporting these experiences, therapists can unravel deeply ingrained patterns, thereby enabling authentic healing.

The enhanced somatosensory sensitivity of the psychedelic state may bring us into contact with our somatic markers. By identifying and documenting these as they arise in the psychedelic journey, we can learn much about the body's primary role in shaping our responses to the world.

Because so much of the inner transformation brought on by psychedelics occurs from the bottom up, the psychedelic therapist must become fluent in the language of the soma. This means building familiarity with interoception and sensing the totality of experience in an integrated gestalt of sensation, image, emotion, and cognition known as the felt sense. The body constantly tries to communicate with us, but these transmissions remain inscrutable until we learn how the body speaks and communicates on *its* terms.

In the next chapter, we explore specific ways of working with bodily responses in therapy, using insights and techniques from somatic modalities.

CHAPTER 4

Somatic Therapies and Expanded States

Embodiment is fundamental to the development of any aspect of a human being.
—SUSAN APOSHYAN

Somatic psychotherapy combines cognitive and emotional therapy with body-centered awareness. In somatic work, body awareness, mindfulness, movement, breathwork, and safe touch are combined with traditional psychotherapeutic tools like dialogue, cognitive and behavioral interventions, and emotional processing.

SOMATIC PSYCHOTHERAPY AND PSYCHEDELICS

Psychedelic experiences highlight nonverbal and physical phenomena, making them quite compatible with somatic therapy. Clinicians who "read" bodily processing will know when to intervene—and when not to. Expanded states of consciousness arise out of embodied consciousness, requiring a clinical skill set beyond conventional talk therapy. If somatic approaches are not included in psychedelic work, the journeyer may be inadequately prepared for the journey.

Clients and research participants often report a strong awareness of their bodies during dosing sessions. After taking these medicines, they report feeling more connected to their somatic selves, accessing new sensations. They may suddenly regain awareness of regions of the body connected to past trauma, or recognize shame as a heaviness in their chest. They may report a profound sense of pleasure in the body: sensations of warmth, tingling, or deep relaxation.

Here are some examples of somatic experiences that can arise with various psychedelic medicines. Each journey is unique, and individuals may have different responses, but certain experiences seem to be common.

MDMA amplifies feelings of empathy and connection, often felt in the body. People become more attuned to the body's need for connection, physically craving proximity with others. Relaxation reduces muscular tension, allowing pleasurable sensations to be more vivid.

Ketamine significantly alters perception of the body. This can result in either dissociation or heightened awareness of bodily sensations. Some clients report out-of-body experiences, in which conscious awareness is somewhere outside of the body, which for some enables them to explore sensations from a different perspective.

Ayahuasca can involve physical purging, often thought to be a cleansing on both physical and emotional levels. Strong visceral sensations draw attention to the body's internal processes.

Psilocybin enhances perception, making physical sensations more vivid and alive. Warping effects are common, with the body seeming to melt. Strong emotions are often felt physically, leading to bodily discharge in the form of crying or laughing.

> *LSD* is often reported to create a feeling of electricity in the body. Sensations described as vivid light coursing through the physical body are commonly reported. There can be a subtle vibratory quality to this, and trembling is not unusual.
>
> *5-MeO-DMT* (O-methylbufotenin) induces particularly intense and varied somatic experiences, often involving powerful energetic surges. The body may fade away, which can be both liberating and disorienting. Like ayahuasca, 5-MeO-DMT may induce purging, along with tingling or vibration.

Somatic therapy can help journeyers navigate the strange and novel sensations that arise on psychedelics. Preparatory somatic work helps clients to trust their bodies and enhances body awareness. Additionally, it gives clients skills to manage experiences, especially under duress.

KEY FEATURES OF SOMATIC PSYCHOTHERAPY

Shaped From the Inside Out

Somatic approaches recognize the interconnectedness of mental, emotional, and physical well-being. We are somatically shaped by the past: family culture, ancestral history, and social influences embedded in the body. Events such as war, famine, systemic oppression, community violence, and intergenerational trauma alter epigenetic mechanisms governing genetic expression (Yehuda & Lehrner, 2018).

Working somatically, we can explore how systemic inequities and historical trauma manifest in our present experience. Our bodies carry the echoes of our ancestors' pain, holding the residue of old traumas—sometimes, from before we were even born—in our bodily memory. Somatic educator Staci Haines (2019) describes this embodied landscape of genetic memory as *sites of shaping*, emphasizing how in therapeutic work these can become *sites of change*. The individual is "impacted by social conditions that break or betray our inherent need for safety, belonging, and dignity" (p. 74). Somatic practitioners tap into awareness of these impacts to uncover pathways for transformation.

Both somatic and psychedelic approaches tap into an implicit understanding, beyond cognition, of how belief systems have shaped us from the inside out. Our mental health challenges are intertwined with our life story, physical health, and how we move through the world. The past shapes our current selves, and this awareness of intersecting influences guides our future development.

Bottom-Up Approach

The bottom-up framing of somatic therapy emphasizes unconscious somatosensory input (Taylor et al., 2010) as the primary avenue for healing and change (rather than verbal processing and cognitive analysis alone). It prioritizes experiential learning over mental understanding or insight, often working with implicit nonverbal memories, involuntary movement, and nervous system responses. Somatic therapists carefully read physiological cues. Impulses to purge, sob, shake, twitch, push, and physically release emotions are all welcome in somatic therapy.

Somatic Intelligence

When grounded in embodiment, our awareness and actions harmonize with our environment, allowing us to engage in more adaptive behavior. Our thoughts and emotions influence physical health—and vice versa—with stress disrupting this delicate balance. Incorporating embodiment practices helps clients tap into their innate resilience, while psychedelic journeys can enhance this awareness and highlight unresolved traumas.

Many people need more skills to observe inner experiences without bias. In today's fast-paced world, we often neglect somatic intelligence, overidentifying with rational thought, which can erode trust in our bodies. Unprocessed emotional traumas contribute to mental and physical distress, especially in cultures that discourage inner listening.

Lifestyle changes and improved relationships are often seen as clients reconnect with their bodies. For example, a journeyer on psilocybin suddenly realized she needed to stop eating sugar and get a medical checkup, leading to the discovery of her prediabetes. Our bodies are constantly sending us messages but we often fail to receive them. A skilled somatic therapist emphasizes body awareness, asking, "How are you feeling in your body right now?" rather than "What does it mean that you feel this way?" This approach encourages deeper somatic listening.

Somatic Awareness

Somatic awareness involves consciously attending to bodily sensations, movements, and expressions. Charlotte Selver, a pioneer in somatic education, defines this as *sensory awareness*—mindfully focusing on present-moment experiences of the body (Selver & Brooks, 2007). This heightened awareness allows for a deep exploration of one's inner experience. Clients develop an internal witness, able to notice the body from inside. Somatic therapists invite clients to notice: "What is your experience at this moment?" No sensations or feelings are ignored, as they all provide valuable information.

Witnessing from the vantage point of somatic awareness helps clients open to unfamiliar and challenging material. Somatic awareness is a key component of MAPS's MDMA treatment protocols for PTSD, encouraging clients to identify and work through what's stuck in the body (Mitchell et al., 2023). It is our perspective that somatic awareness enhances the effectiveness of all therapeutic techniques.

Conscious Breathing

Our breath mirrors our internal state of being. We breathe with our whole body, often unaware that we are in constant metabolic reciprocity with our world. Our health, emotional state, and our trauma history all shape our breathing habits. When we breathe *with* our bodies, we soften. We are present with ourselves as we pay attention to the breath, not trying to control it. A healthy adult takes 12–20 breaths a minute. How many of these are taken consciously? Likely, none! For many people, simply shifting awareness to include the expansion and contraction of the lungs dampens the stress response.

Stanislov Grof, renowned psychiatrist and psychedelic pioneer, codeveloped Holotropic Breathwork with his wife Christina in the 1970s. They discovered that rapid, rhythmic breathing induces a trancelike state that changes brain waves and can induce nonordinary states of consciousness, akin to psychedelic experiences or peak meditative moments. This method of working with the breath can help shift deeply entrenched cognitive habits and enable powerful emotional releases (Grof & Grof, 2023).

Another somatic practice involving breath and movement is Continuum, developed by Emilie Conrad and Susan Harper. Continuum is a gentle practice, which may suit clients who fear the loss of control common to psychedelic experiences. Including subtle breath practices, resonating sounds, and undulating movements, this practice fosters nonordinary awareness and a fluid engagement with the body (Conrad, 1997). Continuum can facilitate direct awareness of one's dynamic inner phenomenology—a crucial aspect of psychedelic therapy.

Somatic Resources

Somatic resources are competencies clients learn to draw upon in vulnerable or stressed moments. Clients can discover their own resources as we explore physical touch, movement, conscious breathing, postural changes, vocal toning, and imagery. Building a set of somatic resources in the preparation phase can help the journey, allowing clients to trust their experience in moments that could feel overwhelming.

They might explore deep breathing for when they're frightened, laying a hand on their belly for when they're nervous, pushing against our hands for when they're angry, or assuming an upright posture to support moving through shame. These physical processes can help steady the choppy waters of a psychedelic journey. The client learns to see their body as a source of strength, a safe place.

Guided inquiry can foster self-discovery. We might ask clients, "How can you be present with this feeling right now?" or "What support do you need to calm your racing breath?" Such investigations empower clients, cultivating agency and self-regulation as they discover their own somatic resources.

Coregulation

In addition to self-regulation, somatic therapy emphasizes *coregulation*: the way two systems can entrain together to regulate alongside each other. Often, this serves as a stepping stone, assisting the client in learning self-regulation. A gentle touch on the arm, a kind gaze, or a moment spent quietly breathing together—all can bring the client's activated system into synchrony with the therapist's, which is hopefully more regulated and can act as a beacon to the client (particularly when they're distressed). In the unpredictable emotional tumult of a psychedelic journey, this may be the practitioner's most powerful intervention.

Sequencing

Sequencing is an approach to establishing safety and building internal resources. The client observes the flow of experience within the body, becoming aware of the connectedness—or *sequence*—of these phenomena, which promotes a sense of coherence and organization. A shift in posture may release tension in a specific area, creating a somatic pathway of change. The discovery of sequences can give clients a blueprint for shifting experiences.

Consider this exchange from a session with one of my [Manuela] clients, illustrating the idea of sequencing:

"When you notice that feeling of release in your belly, what else happens?"

"I feel a sensation of warmth," the client said.

I nodded. "And as you feel that warmth, what does *that* connect to?"

"Like I can handle the fear, that I will be OK."

"With that OK-ness in mind, what do you notice right now?"

"I feel relieved. The fear isn't stopping me right now. I don't feel overwhelmed."

By observing how these patterns flow in sequence, noting where things become stuck—and how they resolve—the therapist identifies connection and disconnection in the body. This provides support for completion and healing. The client's recognition of the natural intelligence revealed in these sequences fosters a deeper sense of coherence.

Slow Processing

We heal when we have the time and space to do so. The body is an organism, and it needs *organismic time*. This concept is congruent with Gestalt therapy, humanistic psychotherapy, and mindfulness-based approaches, which value slower, more expansive rhythms in the therapeutic process.

Our internal perception of past experiences is highly subjective—traumatic events can be as vivid 20 years later as they were yesterday. We can think fast, but our body needs time to metabolize experience. Therefore, somatic therapy is intentionally slow, allowing the nervous system to catch up and integrate unprocessed material. Slowing down can allow conscious recognition of insights that might otherwise get missed. Organismic time aligns with the body's slower processing speed and is an antidote for getting stuck in fight, flight, or freeze reactions.

Somatic Tracking

When traditional foraging peoples hunt animals, they sensitively observe, touch, and sense an animal's path, revealed by its tracks. The imprint of a bear's paw can reveal the creature's size, age, sex, and even mood, giving a clear direction to follow. The tracker's astuteness requires receptivity to information as it is revealed, following clues without judgment or bias.

In somatic therapy, "tracking" is keenly observing the client's moment-to-moment experience, monitoring their posture, breath, and movement with curiosity. Recounting a fearful childhood memory may elicit a small tremor in the client's hands, a sudden sharpness of breath, a flat tone of voice. We closely track these somatic indicators, sometimes mirroring them with our tone, breath, and posture. Clients learn how to track internal states with the therapist's help and guidance.

Under psychedelics, these indicators become more visible. The person's direct experience is exposed, and we can see the body's perspective more clearly. Joining with the client to track a particular movement, a posture, or a vocalization in the journey can help them embody it more, contextualizing what's occurring and potentially revealing deeper meanings. Through this exploration, it may even transform into a somatic resource for the client, a source of healing.

Clearly, somatics has much to offer psychedelic-assisted therapy. In addition to general somatic themes, it's worth emphasizing two established somatic modalities: Hakomi and Somatic Experiencing (SE). They share a nondirective approach and dovetail well with psychedelic work.

HAKOMI MINDFULNESS-CENTERED SOMATIC PSYCHOTHERAPY

The Hakomi method was developed by Ron Kurtz in 1981, combining mindfulness and somatic psychotherapy. The Hopi word "hakomi" translates to "Where do you stand in relation to these many realms?" This embodies an ancient instinct to inquire into the meaning of life. A more modern translation renders this simply as "Who am I?" This phrase encapsulates the essence of the method, an exploration of how each of us structures reality.

Hakomi offers an integrative approach to healing early childhood trauma and psychological, emotional, and relational issues.

Central to Hakomi is facilitating an awareness of each unfolding moment, grounded in five core principles: mindfulness, nonviolence, unity, organicity, and mind–body holism. Hakomi interweaves ancient wisdom with modern psychology, initiating clients into a deeply personal journey of somatic healing.

Hakomi aims to uncover the core organizing beliefs that reside in the mind and manifest in the body. These beliefs often stem from developmentally pivotal life events. Through mindful awareness and relational engagement, the therapist gently reveals core beliefs as they appear in each moment of the client's experience. These beliefs are seen as limitations to fully embodying one's potential. By studying the barriers and protective mechanisms that give rise to unhelpful thinking and dysfunctional behavior, clients can discover new choices and possibilities for healing and growth.

Hakomi emphasizes deep, immersive engagement with internal states, guiding clients toward their inner healing intelligence—a vital ally in the therapeutic process. The therapist helps the client navigate the layered complexity of their inner world within the safe container of the therapeutic relationship.

Hakomi therapists adopt an experimental mindset when working with clients. Through mindful awareness, clients uncover insights, revealing the wisdom underlying their conditioned responses. New perspectives facilitate new choices. With the therapist's skillful guidance toward novel experiences, clients come to understand their original traumas.

Now let's examine each of the Hakomi method's core principles.

The Foundation of Mindfulness

Mindfulness in Hakomi is more than mere observation: It is an active, applied art of attentive presence to the inner dimension of experience. This can include emotion, sensation, mental images, memory, and thought, and it examines how the person organizes their internal world. Mindfulness can be used in both the top-down processing of emotion and cognition and the bottom-up processing of trauma (Ogden et al., 2006). Clients who cultivate awareness of the here and now can better tolerate difficult emotions and sensations.

Mindfulness creates a container of focused, nonjudgmental attention. This allows old narratives to loosen their grip, making nonbiased observation of one's experience possible. Mindfulness practices have been shown to reduce reactivity in the amygdala and promote emotion regulation and better decision making (Davidson et al., 2003). As Kurtz (2015) described, mindfulness is driven by curiosity, enabling clients to engage directly with even the most challenging experiences.

Loving Presence and Nonviolence

The principle of nonviolence is central to Hakomi. The therapist cultivates a "loving presence," imbuing the therapeutic space with safety, acceptance, cooperation, and compassion. This loving presence nurtures the client's openness, guiding them through their own nonlinear healing process. The Hakomi therapist develops a grounded inner presence and listens deeply to the client's essence, following the client's process without pushing or imposing outcomes.

This nonviolent intention creates space for the client's entire being. The Hakomi therapist meets clients where they are, inquiring into their pain and trauma with gentleness and creativity, trusting in the organic unfolding of the healing process. The healing context, characterized by attentive compassion and wisdom, works creatively with the client's resistance to explore habitual patterns.

Acknowledging Unity

Unity in Hakomi, as articulated by Johanson (2015), emphasizes the interconnectedness of our internal landscape, where diverse elements merge into a multifaceted state of being. Through practices that cultivate self-awareness—such as mindfulness—clients perceive their inner world as a unified system. This holistic perspective recognizes every thought, feeling, and physical sensation as inextricably linked, all essential to the therapeutic process. Individual perspectives are viewed within a framework of broader unity that links us to the collective human experience, throughout time and space. The unity principle emphasizes that although we are unique, we are fundamentally interconnected in our shared human struggles. We exist in interdependence with our families and communities and within interconnected systems.

Trusting in Organicity

The principle of organicity recognizes that living systems are inherently self-organizing. Hakomi therapists are attuned to spontaneous shifts and subtle changes within clients, patiently embracing the organic process (Johanson, 2015). Each therapy session becomes a co-created space of creative expression, weaving together unique threads of awareness and learning. Therapists follow the client's natural process, welcoming creative impulses, movements, and emerging insights. This innate impulse for self-correction is revealed in the phrase, "Water knows how to benefit all things without striving" (Johanson & Kurtz, 1991, p. 33). The principle of organicity encourages trust in the natural progression of the healing journey as a form of intelligence.

Integrating the Mind–Body

The principle of mind–body holism emphasizes attention to physical sensations and subtle cues. Through mindful engagement with the body's wisdom, clients can unravel these patterns and transform deeply held narratives from within. This process brings internalized beliefs to consciousness, allowing exploration of the patterns and behaviors that have shaped one's life, fostering the capacity to make new choices. Emotions, as dynamic elements of personal significance, evolve through our ongoing interpretation of experiences (Tronick, 2007).

Exploring the mind–body interface entails deciphering mental imagery, emotions, and sensations, making meaning from experience. This integrated approach empowers clients to rewrite their narratives, promoting healing and personal growth through a deeper understanding of their holistic experience.

SOMATIC EXPERIENCING: A ROAD MAP TO HEALING TRAUMA

Somatic Experiencing® (or, as previously noted, SE™) is a body-centered therapeutic modality developed by Peter Levine. It is a naturalistic approach to the healing and resolution of trauma, and is based on Levine's observations of wild animals. In attempting to understand trauma, he asked, "Why are animals in the wild, though threatened routinely, rarely traumatized?" (Levine, 1997, back cover). He discovered that wild animals have a natural immunity to trauma, and created SE to make this available to people, too. SE has proven efficacy in treating posttraumatic stress (Brom et al., 2017). Harnessing the body's innate capacity for nervous system regulation, SE provides a path for individuals to shake off the residue of past experiences and become more fully alive.

All animals instinctively scan the environment for cues of safety or threat. Novelty is attended to automatically, which Pavlov (1927) called the *investigatory reflex*:

> In a normal animal the slightest alteration in the environment—even the very slightest sound or faintest odour, or the smallest change in intensity of illumination—immediately evokes the reflex which I referred to in the first lecture as the investigatory reflex—"What-is-it?"—manifested by a very definite motor reaction. (p. 29)

We constantly monitor our surroundings, though this usually goes unnoticed.

The default state of the human organism is *relaxed alertness*. Many people who've been traumatized—or who are under chronic stress—are stuck in survival states of fight, flight, or freeze, and their attention reflects hypervigilance or dissociation instead. Becoming oriented, connected to the environment through the senses, can help the organism settle back into relaxed alertness.

SE facilitates oscillation between pleasant and unpleasant experiences, as well as the embodied experience of expansion and contraction accompanying these shifts. Practitioners assist clients in moving from fixity to flow, shifting between nervous system activation and deactivation. SE is bottom up: practitioners work with the nervous system directly to facilitate shifts, creating the conditions in which the organism and psyche can change.

Just as the body heals wounds, the mind is designed to rebound and recover after challenging events. SE empowers individuals to pursue the healing process at a pace that respects their physiological and emotional readiness.

A central feature of this approach is that it helps clients safely complete interrupted self-protective responses, allowing them to move out of the survival states of fight, flight, and freeze. This natural recovery process may include physiological "discharge," such as trembling, crying, laughing, or yawning. SE identifies the tendency of trauma to become "stuck" in the body, resulting in physical and psychological symptoms.

Ultimately, SE practitioners attempt to contact the life force, easing clients back into aliveness. As Peter Levine (personal communication, December 16, 2023) has said, "I don't work with trauma, I work with vitality—and *essence*." This approach is dedicated to awakening a deeper connection with one's authentic being, facilitating the reemergence of the self-organizing tendency in each organism.

Titration

Titration describes the way that—when it comes to trauma—less is more. Levine (2010) borrowed the term from his chemistry background, where it refers to gradually adding one element to another to achieve a desired reaction. Encouraging clients to process trauma incrementally prevents overwhelm, facilitating healing by reintegrating smaller pieces of the experience. This strategy supports gradual integration, processing trauma and stress at a pace that respects their capacity for emotional charge.

Rather than confronting the full intensity of the traumatic event, SE practitioners guide clients through encountering bitesized pieces of the experience. This method enables compressed survival responses to be processed safely, minimizing the risk of overstimulating the nervous system. Practitioners ensure that the client remains within a tolerable range of intensity, avoiding retraumatization.

Pendulation

Pendulation refers to the rhythmic movement between physiological states of expansion and contraction. A natural healing process involves a back-and-forth between activation and deactivation, arousal and settling. Given the right conditions, our innate tendency is to pendulate, fostering equilibrium and resilience.

Unhealed trauma, though, dominates attention, preventing this easy back-and-forth. Many conventional therapies reinforce this by focusing on the details of the traumatic event. Pendulation, though, disrupts the disorganizing pull of traumatic memories, what Levine (2010) called the "trauma vortex."

By helping clients feel how the nervous system spontaneously moves between polarities, mirroring the natural ebb and flow of a wave, balance in the nervous system is restored. SE is oriented toward healing trauma, of all kinds, but more importantly represents the science of how humans can regain our birthright, restoring the intrinsic self-regulatory potential of our organism.

Try This: Conscious Orienting

Encourage your client to connect to the environment regularly. This can be as simple as saying, "Take a moment and let your eyes go where they want to go," but structured orientation techniques can be useful at times. If they feel uneasy or anxious, it can help them ground. Here's a simplified script for practicing orienting:

1. *Assess your state*: Identify how you feel right now. How safe and connected do you feel on a scale of 1–10?
2. *Take a settling breath*: Breathe slowly to center yourself.
3. *Look around*: Start by slowly turning your head and eyes to one side, letting your body follow.

4. *Gentle twist*: Allow yourself to look behind you without straining. Take another settling breath. Go really slow!
5. *Return to center*: Look straight ahead, allowing your eyes to rest without focusing too hard.
6. *Look to the other side*: Repeat the movement on the other side, then return to the center and breathe deeply.
7. *Notice changes*: Reflect on any shifts in your anxiety, vigilance, and breathing.
8. *Relax your eyes*: Look around the room softly, without scanning. Allow your eyes to rest and take in some details. Find something delightful as you look around.
9. *Complete the sequence*: After both sides, return to the center and close your eyes or look down. Check in with your body—do you feel more connected?
10. *Reassess safety*: Take another slow breath. On a scale of 1–10, what is your feeling baseline now? Do you feel calmer, safer, more connected? Write down any observations.
11. *Repeat as needed*: Use this practice whenever you feel anxious or vigilant to help shift those feelings.

INTEGRATING PARTS TOWARD A COHERENT SENSE OF SELF

A common feature of psychedelic work is that clients recognize that they have different aspects of themselves and differing ways of thinking about things and responding to life, which are sometimes called *parts*. Sometimes these parts develop a life of their own, becoming consistent *subpersonalities*, typically developed as protective mechanisms in response to traumatic stress, shame, and other disowned or disavowed elements of experience. In psychedelic states, people commonly see how one part of them thinks or feels one way—while another adopts the opposite perspective. One part may want to be compassionate and open toward others, while another is judgmental and afraid. We may feel loving and angry simultaneously, oscillating between two different vantage points.

Perhaps these various elements of self don't need names or to be reified as distinct personages. Rather than being disturbed by incongruous thoughts or feelings, we can reassure ourselves that it is normal for our inner lives to be a shifting tapestry of experiential states. If we have truly come to know ourselves, we've encountered a host of differing perspectives. The task is to embrace this paradox, letting go of the ego's futile attempt to define the self as a fixed, separate entity. We often cling to the illusion that we can be neatly categorized and predicted, but true understanding requires the acknowledgment of the fluidity of our identity.

These variations in self-identity are revealed during psychedelic journeys. In the preparation session, we can ask clients to identify any disowned parts they're aware of. During the journey, it can be very helpful to facilitate dialogues between different parts, focusing on what it feels like to bodily inhabit each of these selves. Simple invitations like "Allow yourself to be, feel, or move with this part," can serve as a gateway for clients to reconnect with and accept lost aspects of themselves.

Clients may learn to embrace a shame-ridden inner child with unconditional love, facilitating what Hakomi terms a "missing experience": a spontaneous corrective moment absent in past events. Having a felt sense of inner parts can be liberating. This embodied orientation allows clients to relate to their unconscious assumptions in a tangible, nonabstract manner. Parts that are challenging to accept can be approached with greater compassion.

All parts are *us*. By embracing what we have disowned, welcoming our variegated internal experiences, we cultivate a self-concept that is expansive enough to encompass it all.

CONCLUSION

Somatic methods are invaluable tools for psychedelic therapists. These are not mere techniques but a way of being: a warm, nondirective attitude that supports each client's nonlinear unfolding. At the heart of these approaches is a compassionate therapeutic relationship, fostering the emergence of inner wisdom, a knowing that transcends explanation and conscious thought as it catalyzes self-healing. Somatic work registers the silent language of the body and unlocks the full potential of the psychedelic experience.

CHAPTER 5

Adverse Events

Even bad trips, though they can be difficult, can serve as a valuable learning experience.
—HAMILTON MORRIS

I [Joshua] remember visiting my father and stepmother as a preteen, during a school break, and somehow the subject of LSD came up.

"That stuff is *poison*," my stepmother spit out.

She went on to tell a horrific (but surely apocryphal) story, claiming her cousin had taken LSD and then months later experienced a terrifying flashback, committing suicide during the crisis. I now suspect this story was confabulated to ease the grief of the cousin's parents, but it became, to my young mind, the ultimate cautionary tale. An innocent youth in the prime of life had tried a drug for fun, and then out of nowhere, months later, found himself engulfed in a state of madness so encompassing it drove him to end his life. I resolved to stay away from this diabolical drug.

The history of psychedelics is replete with tales like this. Stories of addled teenagers staring at the sun until they go blind—or leaping from buildings believing they could fly—have titillated the public imagination for decades. While these urban legends have in many cases been debunked ("Governor Shafer Calls LSD

Blindings a Hoax"; *The New York Times*, 1968), the true stories never make the front pages. In the public imagination, a question still looms large: What doom awaits me if I dare to take these drugs?

In the current wave of enthusiasm for psychedelic therapy, however, some cheerleaders seem to suggest there's *no* danger. There is a tendency to overcorrect the public image—from evil perversions to angelic saviors, from peril to panacea. This reputational makeover is astonishing, and runs the risk of creating confusion. Here's the truth: Negative outcomes of psychedelic journeys are real, but this need not dim our inspiration for the work. In fact, understanding the potential pitfalls will only make things safer and more effective for journeyers.

SERIOUS AND NONSERIOUS ADVERSE EVENTS

Medical science uses the term "adverse events" to describe undesirable outcomes from a treatment that are not caused by preexisting illness. Any intervention or procedure can have potential *side effects*, impacts outside the scope of treatment that are unwelcome and may exacerbate disease in the brain or body. The outcome can even be *iatrogenic*, meaning that the attempt to heal ends up degrading health: The treatment harms the patient.

It's essential to differentiate between common adverse events and *serious adverse events* (SAEs). In the medical literature, SAEs are adverse events so severe they require hospitalization, or are life-threatening. SAEs are exceedingly rare in psychedelic research, while what we might call non-SAEs—such as physical discomfort or emotional distress—are quite common.

Adverse events—but not SAEs—are intrinsically part of psychedelic work. The majority of journeyers report experiences of feeling frightened, nauseated, sad, hot, and so on. The seasoned psychedelic therapist knows that these phases of adversity are not to be avoided but entered into willingly—or even enthusiastically. When embraced in this way, they often present opportunities for healing. A medical researcher might classify the experience of being moved to tears as an adverse event, but therapeutically speaking this is probably an essential aspect of the healing process.

The way we choose to frame these events can significantly influence the outcome. We don't want to label experience as somehow bad or wrong and create avoidance. If we consider anxiety in the journey to be an "adverse event," clients could end up trying to sidestep difficult feelings. Seeing nausea as a "side effect" of the drug could miss how sickness is one way the body processes emotion and energy. Adversity might be a doorway into deeper healing, requiring openness and acceptance on the part of the journeyer. This requires a reconceptualization of what adverse events in psychedelic work truly are.

That being said, some people experience unmanageable distress in the journey. Psychedelic drugs can create subjective states that are intense, overwhelming, and in some cases traumatizing. We shouldn't flinch from the truth: Some people become damaged—sometimes *badly*—by their psychedelic trip. Thankfully, we can do much to prevent this by screening, preparing, and adequately supporting journeyers through moments of distress.

CHALLENGING EXPERIENCES

Most psychedelic journeys contain periods of adversity. At least transiently, unpleasantness will occur. Psychedelics do not have the soothing quality of alcohol, a central nervous system depressant. Nor do they reliably create euphoric effects like cocaine, stimulating body and mind. Psychedelics may at times mimic the action of other drugs, but are fundamentally unpredictable.

Mood- and mind-altering substances are most often taken for

particular subjective effects. We want to feel a certain way, so we consume the drug most likely to create that state. But psychedelic intoxication is more like rolling the dice. Each journey is unique, and one simply cannot know in advance what the unconscious has in store, or how the conscious mind will respond.

Even the most experienced journeyers, with the best support, sometimes have "bad trips." While there has been a recent trend to reframe these negative journeys as *challenging experiences*—a shift in language intended to help people relate differently to adversity—no one can deny that they are profoundly unpleasant, and may even cause lasting psychological damage.

Some people report that challenging experiences can be just as therapeutic as pleasant journeys, though. Working through these negative experiences in the integration phase, investigating the neuroses and mental fixations they reveal, has led some to boldly affirm that there *are* no bad trips, that everything in the journey can be grist for the mill.

An unresolved bad trip, however, may increase the likelihood that we'll have bad trips in the future. Citing Hemsley and Ward, Aixalà (2022) writes, "The occurrence of difficult psychedelic experiences in the past appears to be a significant predictor of their repetition" (p. 35).

Carbonaro et al. (2016) found that 39% of subjects rated their "worst bad trip" as one of the five most challenging experiences of their lives. This should sensitize us to the seriousness of challenging experiences. However, it's important to note that in this same study, the majority of respondents indicated that the degree of acute difficulty in the journey was associated with eventual increases in well-being. In other words, those who suffered the most in their journeys reported more enduring shifts in their day-to-day lives. Does this mean that suffering in a journey is inherently good? No. At the same time, the psychedelic therapist should recognize that challenges successfully met build resilience. Facing one's demons can be liberating. Again, knowing when (and how) to intervene is what's key.

INTERVENING IN ADVERSE EVENTS

A crucial finding from research on adverse events reported in psychedelic studies is that *longer duration and greater severity of distress predict more negative outcomes* (Carbonaro et al., 2016; Roseman et al., 2018). Therefore, therapists need to be prepared to intervene, sometimes vigorously, to make sure journeyers don't get stuck in adversity. And it happens that some of the best interventions available come from somatic therapy. Peregrine Somerville (personal communication, June 28, 2024), an SE practitioner and licensed psilocybin facilitator in Oregon, relates this account:

> The first psilocybin journey I ever guided in a licensed service center was for my practicum—the final phase of my facilitator training, and a requirement for state licensure. My client was a classmate, a young man with whom I'd built some rapport throughout the training; 18 milligrams was a comparable dose to what he'd taken in previous journeys, but this time it hit him far harder than he was expecting.
>
> It was winter in Portland, late afternoon and the light through the western windows was fading. As the administration room steadily darkened, the music darkened with it. The playlist—a creation of my supervisor, unfamiliar to me—was loud in the speakers overhead, the layers of minor key strings clashing together in a weird, warbling overtone. The song was ominous, disorienting, and I was *sober*.

My client had stayed internal through the come-up, laid out on a mat under eye mask and headphones. Now he sat up and raised the mask. His brow furrowed, face pale with fear.

"Are we . . . *okay* here?" he said, darting his eyes around the shadowed room.

"Okay here?" I said, careful to keep my tone neutral.

"Yeah. Like, are we *safe* here? Is this a *safe place* to be?"

"Yes, we're good here. You are completely safe in this place."

He nodded, lowered the mask, and lay back down. A moment later he was up again.

"It's just that . . . I'm not *totally sure* . . . that I'm safe right now." He grimaced, jaw clenching, his face strained with worry. "It's really dark in here," he said. "And it's getting darker."

I swallowed. I knew he wasn't just talking about the room. His journey was taking a dark turn and he was afraid for his safety. "And are you . . . able to be with that darkness?" I asked.

He drew a sharp breath, shook his head. "No, I—I don't actually think I can."

My heart lurched. I realized with a shock that my facilitator training had done nothing to prepare me for this moment. All the neurobiology lectures, the intake roleplays, the social equity workshops, the quizzes on state regulations, but they'd given me no tools for redirecting a bad trip, not a single one. I sat there in stunned silence as he trembled with the mounting panic. He'd warned me of his tendency to get sucked into thought loops, endless cycles of self-centralized dread. Now it was happening. I could see hours passing in this way—the paranoid fantasies enflaming his mind as his body flooded with cortisol, his intention for the journey receding into the distance.

He gave me a pleading look. Opened his mouth to speak, but no words came.

I'd asked him if he could be with it, if he could abide in this darkness. He'd told me no. And so, without any conscious intent, I reached for my somatics toolkit.

"Want to come with me over to the window?" I said.

He frowned. "The window?"

"Yeah. Let's go sit together by the window for a minute. Come on."

Outside the sky was ashen. Clouds clung to the tops of buildings downtown, as the steely gray Willamette River snaked beneath the city's long chain of bridges. "What do you see?" I asked.

"That bird." He pointed to a lone seagull gliding on an updraft.

"Nice. And what do you notice about that bird?"

"It's just hanging tough," he said. "The wind kicks up, it gets blown around a bit, then the wind dies back down, and it's not bothered by any of it. Doesn't even flap its wings. It's just hanging out."

"Great. And as you notice that it's just hanging out, what do you experience inside?"

He closed his eyes. His arms floated out to either side. "It's like something's holding me up."

"Like something is holding you up. Can you just be with that feeling for a moment?"

He nodded, arms hovering in the air. The corner of his mouth twitched up a hair. Then he drew a deeper breath, let it sigh away, and his eyes opened. There was a softness to them I hadn't seen all day.

I smiled. "What else are you seeing out here?"

"That kayaker." He pointed to a man in blue rain gear, floating downriver in a kayak.

"What do you notice about that kayaker?"

"He . . . he isn't paddling. His oar's laid across his lap. He's just going with the current."

"Beautiful. And as you notice that he's just going with the current, what do you feel inside?"

Again he closed his eyes. One hand alighted on his chest, the other on his belly. "I can feel my breath filling me, keeping me afloat. It's like I can just go with the current. I know I'm not going to drown." He opened his eyes, looked at me. "You know, I think I'm ready to lie back down."

I followed him across the room to his mat, helped him get situated with his eye mask and headphones, crossed his arms over his chest, and let out a quiet sigh of relief. It was a simple intervention, a technique from my SE training—oscillating attention externally and internally in a steady rhythm until the client's activation abates—but it had worked. Thankfully, those were the only choppy waters we had to navigate that day. As I watched over him in the next few hours of relative calm, I found myself wondering, what if I hadn't known the Somatic Experiencing method? What if the only skills I had available were from my facilitator training? What on earth would I have done then?

There are many possible interventions when a journey starts spiraling downward. The therapist can change an element of the *setting*, such as switching the music to something lighter and more uplifting, rearranging the lighting concept in the room, or taking the journeyer outside or on a walk. In extreme cases, pharmacological interventions may be employed: "aborting" a trip with antipsychotic drugs or benzodiazepines, if this is within one's scope of practice.

What makes the above example so illustrative, though, is that the therapist chose to intervene on the level of *set*. He redirected the journeyer's focus of attention away from the anxiety and paranoia, thereby shifting the contents of consciousness to external and internal percepts that were less threatening. It would be tempting to label this as a distraction. In fact, though, the oscillation of the client's awareness—outward, then inward, then outward again—created enough distance from the fear that he could metabolize it, readying him to return inside again (see "The Monster in the Mirror" section in Chapter 6). Remember, it *matters* what journeyers pay attention to, and they have more agency in this than they may realize. In moments when they're unable to redirect attention on their own, we are there to help them.

DETERMINANTS OF ADVERSE EVENTS

Skillfully tailoring one's therapeutic style to each journeyer requires knowing when (and when not) to intervene. This could be related to their personality characteristics. It has been found that people high in the personality traits of absorption, openness, and acceptance tend to have more positive outcomes, while those low in these features—or who find themselves in a preoccupied or apprehensive state beforehand—have more negative outcomes (Aday et al., 2021). We can assess the journeyer's traits and tendencies in the preparation phase, recognizing those for whom a more interventionist approach may be necessary.

Traits describe predictable patterns of response, while *states* are passing experiences. People low in trait *absorption*—a predisposition to become engrossed in the contents of experience—may resist psychedelic effects. The same goes for people low in trait *openness*—receptivity to new ideas and experiences. This is not to suggest that such individuals will automatically have an adverse event occur in the dosing session. But the therapist will need to ease them into accepting the altered state, encouraging them to "go with the flow" of the journey.

It may also become necessary for we therapists to remind *ourselves* to go with the flow of the journey. A client's suffering in session will impact us, and our habitual responses to suffering can then influence their experience, potentially in ways that may not be helpful.

Try This: Responses to Suffering

Briefly recall an interaction with a client, one where they became visibly upset in session. When the client broke down in tears or expressed anger, did you feel relieved that they were finally getting "real"? Did you coax them toward the feeling, so the pain could be felt as deeply as possible? Or did you instead feel a need to end their suffering, offer them a different way of framing the problem, or remind them of something positive? Do you tend to see the suffering of your clients as something to be entered into fully, or something to be transcended and overcome?

Observe what your typical response is, and try not to judge it. We all have our habitual reactions to the suffering of others, informed by our own histories and personalities. The next time this happens in session, experiment with *not* reacting, not saying anything. Simply direct your gaze in their direction, beaming with compassion and curiosity. Or ask open-ended, value-neutral questions. Try to adjust your internal posture, creating enough space inside yourself for their inner healer to come forward.

DOSAGE

Another key influence on adverse events is dosage. Unsurprisingly, a higher dose has been shown to create more dysphoric effects (Griffiths et al., 2011; Holze et al., 2020). As mentioned, Grof (1980) called psychedelics "unspecific amplifiers" (p. 52). Taking psychedelics in massive doses is like—as Spiñal Tap always did—turning the amplifier up to 11 (Reiner, 1984). Any negativity or pain lurking in the mind may rampage into awareness with a vengeance, leading to more challenging and difficult-to-integrate experiences.

Journeyers often report that the higher the dose, the less ability they have to "steer" the flow of the journey, or make decisions. Put another way, more drugs equals less agency. This total loss of control may allow for powerful experiences of release and surrender, but can just as easily result in feelings of overwhelming helplessness. Dosage must be carefully considered, targeted to the specific personality traits, expectations, and capacities each client has.

That being said, a truly dangerous overdose of psychedelics would be difficult to achieve. The LD_{50} (lethal dose for 50% of an experimental animal population) of psilocybin is 280 milligrams per kilogram (2.2 pounds) of body weight (Cerletti, 1958, as cited in Passie et al., 2002). This would be 22.4 grams of pure psilocybin for an average American, meaning the amount required to kill a human being is roughly *700 times* a usual therapeutic dose. That's a lot of mushrooms! So, while it's somewhat easy to take a dose of psychedelics that is "too much" to psychologically tolerate, it's quite a challenge to take a dose that is physically unsafe. Nevertheless, dosage should be monitored carefully for each client.

ADDICTION

Addressing adverse events around drug dosage necessitates a discussion of addiction. Psychedelics are widely understood to be nonaddictive. Their subjective effects can be *dysphoric*, or emotionally unpleasant, so people do not tend to use them habitually. Tolerance builds quickly, making it difficult to maintain a daily habit of psychedelic use. People often report needing twice as much the next day to attain the same high. There is also cross-tolerance between the classic psychedelics, meaning that someone who had just used LSD would require a larger dose of psilocybin—and vice versa (this applies to mescaline as well).

If one somehow developed a regular psychedelic habit, taking an ever-increasing dose, stopping would not result in withdrawal symptoms, and no physiological cravings would occur. Psychological dependence is also rare, making it even less likely one could develop a true addiction. Rather than presenting an addiction risk, data suggest we should be looking to psychedelics as a possible *treatment* for addiction (van der Meer et al., 2023).

PHYSIOLOGICAL ADVERSE EVENTS

There is a wide range of adverse physiological effects that a client may experience during or after their journey. All of these possible effects should be mentioned in the written consent form(s) that the client signs during the preparation stage. Some clients experience headaches in their journey. Although psychedelics are currently being researched as a treatment for cluster headache (Schindler et al., 2024), alongside other complex pain syndromes (Robinson et al., 2024), people regularly report pain in their head during or after their journey. Clients should be prepared for this, particularly if they tend to get headaches in response to stress.

Certain clients will feel nauseated. Some of these agents will agitate the digestive system, especially if the journeyer has an empty stomach. Also, for whatever reason, some people respond to experiential intensity with nausea, and coming up on psychedelics elicits this response. Preparing clients for this, and letting them know that feeling queasy can be explored like any other sensation, can allow for a nonreactive and nonjudgmental tolerance of nausea. Some journeyers discover that their sickness has an emotional component, facilitating deeper processing.

Fatigue is very common, sometimes during the journey itself but more often afterward. Clients often feel "wiped out" the next day(s), and ideally should clear their schedule for recovery and integration work. The transition into and out of expanded states is tiring, mentally and physically, and though their existential outlook may be transformed, clients will rarely feel energized following a journey.

Because psychedelics—and especially MDMA—have sympathomimetic effects, it is common for heart rate and blood pressure to be elevated. This may feel unpleasant, and can induce a sense that something is wrong. Clients attending to their bodies may be alarmed by how fast, or hard, their heart is beating. However, this physiological reaction is not necessarily related to the client's trauma or unconscious material. Remember, physical phenomena can sometimes reflect unconscious emotional processing, but sometimes it's just the body being affected by a powerful material. The therapist can remind clients that tachycardia—elevated heart rate—is a known effect of the drug, and may very well have nothing to do with their underlying emotional state. The consent form(s) should include a place for the client to disclose any heart condition that might be aggravated by psychedelics.

In Chapter 3, we discussed how somatic markers can be a doorway into working with emotions. Sometimes, though, we may need to remind journeyers that organs in the body are affected by substances, too, and that this may not mean anything in particular. It could be helpful to direct attention away from that somatic experience rather than exploring it, particularly if it's causing undue distress.

A common side effect of MDMA (and some classic psychedelics) is bruxism—jaw clenching or teeth grinding. This is a behavior we would find highly relevant in regular therapy sessions. In body-centered psychotherapy, for instance, tension in the jaw could mean that the person needs to process anger or is bracing against experience. But again, MDMA simply makes jaws clench, and this is not necessarily a symptom of an underlying affect.

On ayahuasca, journeyers should expect vomiting (and sometimes diarrhea). In the shamanic traditions of Central and South America, these expulsions are seen as part of the cleansing power of the medicine, sometimes referred to as "getting well." The body purging itself is regarded as therapeutic, a release of accreted psychospiritual sickness. If vomiting occurs, on any of the psychedelics, it could be useful for the therapist to introduce the possibility that expelling the contents of the stomach is healing. Clients can actively participate in this process by inquiring into which "sickness" is being purged, as is common practice in shamanic traditions.

We should stress that none of the aforementioned physiological responses are intrinsically harmful. Although psychedelics radically transform perceptions, cognitions, and emotions, bodily functions tend to remain within the normal range. In fact, it is remarkable that these substances alter psychological experience so dramatically while impacting physiology so little. Usually, mind and body are best understood as an integrated entity, a psychophysiological unity in which change in one presupposes change in the other. However, psychedelics seem to be unique in their capacity to drastically alter neurological processes without significantly shifting the function of organs and glands.

Simply put, the classical psychedelics rarely impact physical health in a negative way. Of course, this doesn't suggest that the experience is benign, and psychedelic therapists should carefully consider the various risks these drugs present. Let us always recall the words from the Hippocratic oath: "I will do no harm." This is the principle of *non-maleficence*—the helper makes sure they are not hurting before attempting to heal. Psychedelic therapy requires this commitment, perhaps more than most treatment approaches. A bad psychedelic experience can be ruinous. We must exercise caution around how—and with whom—we administer these substances.

EXISTENTIAL THREATS

Adverse events on psychedelics can include existential threats, such as the feeling that one is dying. Journeyers may be unable to perceive their own vital functions, or simply have a strong foreboding that the end is near. This primordial fear can lead clients into recurrent cycles of biting panic. However, it's important to note that *dying before dying* is recognized by many spiritual traditions as a key to living fully. A symbolic or metaphorical death can be thought of as preparation for one's eventual literal death, and the psychedelic therapist can encourage trust and openness to this provocation. Grof (1980) identified this as central to the change process: "The main objective of psychedelic therapy is to create optimal conditions for the subject to experience the ego death and the subsequent transcendence into the so-called psychedelic peak experience" (p. 35), "... which usually takes the form of a death–rebirth sequence with ensuing feelings of cosmic unity" (p. 37). Stories of psychological death and symbolic dismemberment abound in shamanic initiations around the world. We can trust that the self will be put back together in a more coherent fashion after it endures being rent asunder.

Of course, if the journeyer doesn't have the ego strength to abide this ultimate fear, or if the distress continues on for too long, it is useful to coax them away from the belief that they're dying. The therapist can remind the client that they've taken a drug, that this reaction is common, and it's illusory. Invite them to feel into their living body, and remember they're actually fine.

Another existential threat that may arise is the fear of going crazy. Though acutely painful, this transitory crisis may be an opportunity to reclaim a disowned aspect of the psyche.

Turning toward these monstrous fears, the most basic terrors that torment us—ceasing to *be*, or ceasing to be *me*—can open us to glorious moments of transcendent illumination. People may discover that there is something beyond the incessant clinging to life, or maintaining rigid control of the mind, something far more expansive and freer. Again, though, the therapist will at times need to reassure journeyers. They can confidently, perhaps even nonchalantly, convey that the fear of madness is a common response to these drugs, and not worth worrying about.

CHALLENGES AFTER JOURNEYS

Clients sometimes experience enduring distress in the aftermath of a psychedelic journey. Profound openings of the psyche, if not well contained, can challenge the journeyer's ability to stabilize afterward. Journeyers may report feeling spacey, adrift, ungrounded, or anxious, for days, weeks, or even months after a potent experience.

It is worth noting that meditation teachers also face this problem, as periods of intensive retreat practice can evoke many of the same responses. Any initiation into expanded states often leaves a person shaky afterward, and this could be read as part of a larger healing process. Integration sessions will be helpful, including assurances that this is normal and not to be feared.

A psychotic break can also occur after a psychedelic journey. This is exceedingly rare, but again, such adverse events must be acknowledged and contended with. In 1960, Cohen examined the large body of existing literature on psychedelic therapy, finding that only one subject out of 1,200 showed a psychotic reaction that lasted more than 48 hours (as cited in Schlag et al., 2022). Importantly, this individual was the identical twin of a schizophrenic sibling, and would have been screened out of current research protocols (and the offices of most psychedelic therapists).

Still, any client may need some kind of psychiatric attention in the aftermath of a journey. It is part of the therapist's responsibility to make sure that their client is relatively stable before releasing them from the session. Still feeling "high" after the acute drug effects have worn off isn't unheard of. Clients may be alarmed as their mind continues to function in unfamiliar ways, even after the point they expected to have "come down." Labeling this as psychosis may be premature, or outright false. Generally, these reactions abate within a day or two.

As Western society recovers from decades of fearmongering about psychedelics, there remains widespread concern about their danger to our minds. It could be corrective, then, to look at an enormous, nationwide study of drug use and its impacts on mental health. A randomly selected sample of 135,095 Americans (including 19,299 psychedelic users) found no link between psychedelic use and mental health disorders (Johansen & Krebs, 2015). Rather, it found that those who had used psychedelics—in any context, at any point in their lives—were *less* likely than other drug users to have utilized mental health services in the preceding year.

AFTERGLOW

Sometimes adverse events in a journey can lead to catharsis—the release of pent-up emotions and the processing of painful sensations and dark thoughts. These releases can be healing, even if the journey itself is hard. A commonly reported effect of psychedelics is the *afterglow*, a feeling of freshness or goodness in the day(s) after a journey.

Albert Hofmann (1980), renowned chemist and pharmacological innovator, took the first acid trip in 1943 after synthesizing LSD in his lab. The experience terrified him. He described LSD as "the demon that scornfully triumphed over my will," and wrote that he was "seized by the dreadful fear of going insane" (p. 18). However, the morning following this first acid trip he experienced the acid afterglow: "A sensation of well-being and renewed life flowed through me . . . the world was as if newly created. All my senses vibrated in a condition of highest sensitivity, which persisted for the entire day" (p. 19). Actually, some regular psychedelic users have reported a stronger afterglow following challenging experiences, as if the strength of the *glow* reflects a purging of unconscious psychic material.

FLASHBACKS AND HALLUCINOGEN-PERSISTING PERCEPTION DISORDER

Other aftereffects of psychedelic use include *flashbacks*—a recurrence of the psychedelic state without drug administration. This mysterious phenomenon has perplexed observers for decades, with spurious theories introduced to explain it. Some speculated that errant molecules of the drugs were stored in fatty tissues and suddenly released, while others alleged that the substances lurked forever in the spinal fluid of users, intruding on the brain at unpredictable moments. These are urban legends, of course. Whatever flashbacks are, they are not the result of drugs magically stored in the body. As experiences in meditation, ritual, and trance show, the brain is entirely capable of manufacturing its own expanded state of consciousness. Why this occurs for some psychedelic users afterward is unknown.

When flashbacks persist and cause clinically significant distress, they can meet criteria for *hallucinogen-persisting perception disorder* (HPPD), introduced in the American Psychiatric Association's (APA; 2013) fifth edition of the *Diagnostic and Statistical Manual of Mental Disorders* (*DSM-5*). This psychiatric bible reports the prevalence of HPPD as 4.2% of psychedelic users (APA, 2013), though this figure was deduced from a single online questionnaire (Baggott et al., 2011). In 1979, Grinspoon and Bakalar aggregated data available at that time to come up with an estimate of 1 HPPD sufferer in 50,000 psychedelic users. If the actual prevalence of HPPD is around 1 in 25, instead—as the *DSM-5* claims—we would expect current psychedelic research to have generated many, many cases. However, among thousands of participants in dozens of studies there are no reports of HPPD (Schlag et al., 2022). Perhaps this reflects proper screening and preparation. Or maybe HPPD is rarer than the APA thought.

Additionally, many people who *do* experience flashbacks report these unexpected shifts into altered states to have a neutral—or even positive—valence (Müller et al., 2022). Changes in visual perception or affective tone can be appreciated as delightful surprises, or they may be interesting but unremarkable. We shouldn't assume that nonordinary states of consciousness, even when unexpected, are inherently aversive.

One interesting hypothesis is that HPPD is a form of posttraumatic stress. Halpern et al. (2018) found that among 19 individuals with HPPD, all of them had panic or significant anxiety during the psychedelic experience. In fact, Grof (1980) opined that flashbacks reflect something incomplete, or unmetabolized, in the psychedelic experience. Clients suffering from HPPD may need support to process through their past journey, potentially reentering the psychedelic state with the right guidance to work through what's still incomplete.

SUICIDAL THOUGHTS

Another type of adverse event that may occur in the aftermath of a journey is suicidal ideation. Some people get depressed after a psychedelic experience. Having reached into the beyond, coming back to day-to-day banalities can feel meaningless. The unconscious may have revealed that the journeyer has settled for inadequate marriages or jobs, and dissatisfaction with one's life circumstances is not uncommon. This reorganization of priorities is often overwhelming and confusing, and the inability to affect immediate change in one's life may create hopelessness. Ending one's life can seem like an appropriate solution, though these feelings are most often transitory. Integration sessions will be critical here. We discuss how to best support clients through crises of meaning in the Post-Journey Work section, but for now can just say that it's a type of adverse event some have to live through.

Given all of these potentials for negative outcomes, more research into adverse events and how to treat them is necessary.

Evans et al. (2023) solicited questionnaire data from people who reported ongoing issues after psychedelic use. Of the 608 respondents who were suffering from symptoms after their psychedelic experience (not necessarily undertaken with a therapist or guide), roughly one third of them had distress that lasted over 1 year, while one sixth had suffered over 3 years. This kind of ongoing suffering is a possible outcome of psychedelic use, making it crucially important that preparation and guiding are continually refined to reflect our current understanding of best practices. It is also noteworthy, though, that—even among this cohort—most respondents continued to affirm the value of psychedelic experiences. In fact, 89.7% of respondents agreed with the following statement: "I believe that the insights and healings gained from psychedelics, when taken in a supportive setting, are worth the risks involved."

CONCLUSION

For anyone interested in preparing journeyers, holding space for psychedelic experiences and/or supporting integration, an understanding of adverse events is crucial. Given an optimal set and setting with the right supports, psychedelic journeys are often a provocative catalyst for healing and transformation. However, adverse events are to be expected, prepared for, normalized, and integrated afterward. This work is not for the faint of heart.

CHECKLIST: ADVERSE EVENTS

People may have adverse reactions when coming into contact with psychedelics. We want prospective journeyers to be informed about these risks:

- ☐ The onset of the altered state can feel very provocative, with the first 30–60 minutes being characterized by transient waves of anxiety as the effects take hold.
- ☐ Temperature fluctuations are common, with the body alternating between cold and hot.
- ☐ Nausea, particularly when coming up on the drug, is normal.
- ☐ Heart rate will be increased, which can be scary for some people.
- ☐ Particularly if the session includes MDMA, bruxism (jaw clenching) is very likely.
- ☐ Particularly with ayahuasca, purging (vomiting and/or diarrhea) is usual.
- ☐ Many people experience a feeling of urinary urgency, without being able to urinate.
- ☐ Intense imagery, powerful emotions, and sudden, startling insights are to be expected throughout the journey.
- ☐ Some people have a challenging experience (colloquially called a "bad trip"), in which recurrent cycles of panic, rage, or paranoia can be felt. This ends when the drug effects wear off, but can be difficult to integrate.
- ☐ Some people will feel intensely afraid of going crazy, or dying.
- ☐ Though rare, a full-blown psychotic reaction can occur after exposure to psychedelics.
- ☐ Headache is not uncommon, sometimes during the experience but more often afterward.
- ☐ Fatigue is to be expected, especially on the day(s) following the journey. Sleep disturbance is not at all unusual.
- ☐ Some people have flashbacks: transient, random recur-

rences of psychedelic effects. Infrequently, this persists and becomes long term.

- ☐ At times, the journeyer may have trouble relating to others, even friends and family members they've known for years.
- ☐ Some people can feel depressed afterward, even experiencing a desire to commit suicide. This is rare for people who've never felt that before, but not unheard of.

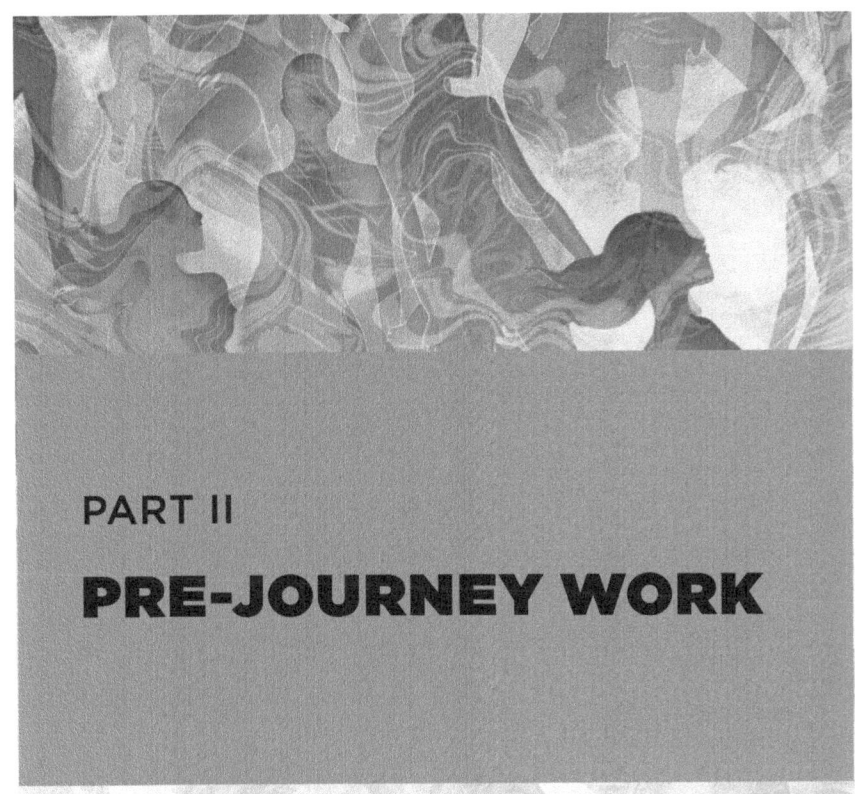

PART II
PRE-JOURNEY WORK

CHAPTER 6

Preparing the Therapist

The therapist's inner experience is the most important tool in the therapeutic process.
—IRVIN D. YALOM

As therapists, we cannot expect to help others—even with the aid of psychedelics—if we haven't embarked on our own healing journey. It's not necessary to be "done" with our work before addressing clients' needs—after all, the journey never ends. But we must recognize the interrelatedness of helping others and our own healing.

When we think of preparation, what typically comes to mind is gathering information from the client and setting up the journey space. What needs equal attention, though, is preparing the therapist's state of being. We need to ready ourselves to attend to the client's energetic shifts, psychic openings, and the traumas that may emerge.

Psychedelic sessions can be emotionally draining, and require multiple hours of sustained presence. The intensity of this work requires more attention than standard therapy, lasting significantly longer than the 50-minute session many practitioners are accustomed to. To skillfully sit and hold space, we must train ourselves in the subtleties of embodied presence and compassion.

This requires work and dedication. In this chapter we explore the process of preparation for the psychedelic therapist.

THE INNER STATE

The bodily state of the therapist is a critical part of set and setting. Again, we tend to think of set as the intention and psychological readiness of the journeyer, while setting describes the environment in which the journey occurs. Actually, though, the internal state of the therapist is the foundation on which the client's experience is built. How the therapist feels inside, the kind of attention they bring to the work, and their level of embodiment all contribute to the quality of the psychedelic session. We could think of this as our *somatic set*: the way we inhabit our bodies as we hold space for others.

Let's look at an example of the failure to tend to set and setting. In a dual-therapist session, the attending psychiatrist, a White man, came in late to the dosing session and was visibly unprepared and mentally frazzled. The client, a Middle Eastern woman, was nervous but excited about her first psychedelic experience. The psychiatrist hurried through the ketamine protocol and expectations for the session. The other attendant, a psychotherapist, observed the client's body becoming increasingly tense, shoulders creeping up to her ears, her posture collapsed. The tension in the room was palpable. The more the psychiatrist bombarded the client with information, the more anxious the client became. He was "doing his job"—but neglected to put himself in compassionate attunement with a vulnerable person facing an unknown experience.

He told the client not to worry, and assured her he'd expertly conducted many of these sessions. Yet the client's bodily response revealed how disturbed she felt. The psychiatrist's callousness and his bravado as a medical expert triggered her early traumatic memories of racism and cultural exclusion. Her journey was starting from a dark place.

As the ketamine session progressed, he became distracted, checking emails as he scrolled through the music playlist. The client's experience reflected both the instability of the environment and the scattered attention of the psychiatrist. Grasping for any semblance of control and safety, her tense body resisted the process and she could not let go into the journey. In the aftermath of the dosing session she felt shrunken, disconnected, and depleted.

In the integration session, the therapist team did nothing to acknowledge the impact of their lack of presence. When the client named that she had not felt fully safe, they reframed this as resistance to the work. The therapists seemed to have no awareness of their influence on her state of mind and the quality of her experience. It was all construed as the client's fault.

SOMATIC SET AND SETTING

So, how can we prevent such neglectful and potentially damaging sessions? The key is for the therapist to establish the proper somatic set. How we *are* in our soma—calm or agitated, present or distracted—impacts the state of the client and the character of their experience. Most clients are anxious, or at least a little nervous, when they begin their journey. They need to meet a stable nervous system with which they can coregulate.

Humans implicitly seek safety by tracking cues from speech patterns, movements, gestures, and facial expressions. In fact, research suggests that the majority of human communication is nonverbal (Mehrabian, 1971). The meaning we derive from any communication is significantly influenced by extralinguistic information: the story that another person's posture, tone of voice, and movements convey.

We don't establish trust with words alone, and we know almost instantly when we don't feel safe. Quick judgments about a face's trustworthiness, likability, and aggressiveness are made in as little as 100 milliseconds (Willis & Todorov, 2006). Research has shown that seeing angry faces—even if the exposure isn't consciously recognized—makes our own facial muscles activate (Dimberg et al., 2000). We also see activation in a brain region called the amygdala, which is associated with the stress response, when unconsciously exposed to fearful faces (Morris et al., 1998). Safety is communicated nonverbally from body to body, so rapidly that we're not even aware of it.

This automatic assessment of safety is called *neuroception* by psychophysiology pioneer Stephen Porges (2022). Neuroception emphasizes that this perception is happening below the level of conscious awareness, that it's an instinctually based *neuro*logical per*ception*. This trait is shared across species, allowing animals to react immediately to perceived threats without thinking. Primed to detect these subtle cues, we respond physiologically by accelerating or decelerating the stress response—according to how we perceive the environment and its inhabitants. For example, friendly eye contact may make our body take a deeper, fuller breath, or a soothing voice can invite our body to relax. Conversely, a person making sharp, erratic movements, or darting their eyes around the room, may signal our palms to sweat and our throat to tighten. We constantly respond to neuroceptive cues physiologically, which shapes our emotional state and our responses to others.

In expanded states, somatosensory processing becomes heightened—and neuroception may be sensitized. If the therapist is distracted or upset, the client may feel internally distressed—without necessarily knowing why. The client's unconscious assessment of safety—or lack thereof—can determine whether they befriend the experience, surrendering into the expanded state with curiosity and wonder, or fight against it.

In indigenous ayahuasca traditions, the body and mind are cleansed through a restrictive diet and sequence of ritual preparations. Being *clean*, in these approaches, refers to both a mindset and a physical purification, preparing one to enter the sacred realm of this medicine. Many Indigenous guides don ceremonial clothing, carry particular ritual objects, paint their faces and bodies, and perform sacred songs to mark the transition from the ordinary world into expanded realms. The guide becomes a vessel for the work, aligning themselves with their lineage of healing. This prepares the practitioner to be in service of the sacred journey.

In the psychedelic therapy office, you can mark the transition into expanded states with the same kind of intention. Some therapists have Indigenous teachers who have permitted them to utilize particular rituals with clients—though if they are not from those traditions themselves, this requires a high degree of cultural sensitivity. We can discover our own traditions, too. Perhaps there is a piece of jewelry or clothing you put on only when guiding journeys, a song you sing or a prayer you recite before the journeyer arrives, or sitting in meditation to open and sensitize your awareness. Certain practices are reported to be especially beneficial: *metta* cultivates loving-kindness through internally wishing others well; in *tonglen*, we imagine taking in the suffering of others and offering back peace and well-being. There are infinite forms of sacred preparation for the psychedelic journey. Find the practices that genuinely speak to you.

THE MULTIDIMENSIONAL THERAPIST

When we assume our role as therapist, we meet ourselves where we are, nonjudgmentally aware of ourselves and the client. We bring an attitude of expertise and professionalism leavened with curiosity and humility. We exude confidence, ready to meet whatever arises and receptive to whatever appears.

Our confidence doesn't come from a place of ego. Rather, it is a kind of compassionate fearlessness. Being multidimensional means, in part, that we are centered, self-assured, and emotionally available to the client. All of these seemingly disparate dimensions of being are alive in us when we hold this seat.

Unconditioned confidence needs to be trained. We cannot simply think ourselves into this state of basic trust; it is an embodied sense developed through lived experience.

Take a moment to recall a mentor or teacher who embodied this kind of confidence, remembering how you felt in their presence. Chances are, you felt safe without thinking about it; it just felt right. Perhaps, in proximity to them you felt a sense of comfort, or an assurance that you could meet the unknown.

The psychedelic-assisted therapist must also cultivate a capacity to hold multiple dimensions of being. We need to be ethical, grounded, competent, compassionate, humble, open, and easygoing, as we navigate some of the most challenging conditions of the human psyche. We must open our awareness to the sensorial field, extending attentive curiosity in all directions.

Try This: Multidimensional Breathing

This practice supports you in becoming multidimensional, attending to the subtle energetic shifts within yourself and the client at the same time.

Take a comfortable standing position, allowing your arms to hang loosely by your sides. Feel your breath in the center axis of your body. As you exhale, imagine that the breath is moving out in all directions from the center of your body into the space around you. Slowly raise your arms out to either side, extending awareness horizontally with your palms down. Follow the breath from your core all the way to your fingertips—and then beyond. Inhale naturally and relax into the standing posture, allowing yourself to be recharged with breath. If your eyes are closed, open them and gaze gently into the space without grasping at anything you see.

Now, imagine your body expanding from your core, breathing outward beyond the periphery of your skin into boundless space around you. Soften your gaze as you extend your spatial awareness. Rest in your standing posture. Slowly return your arms to rest and let them hang loosely by your sides, allowing your eyes to remain open. How do you perceive yourself now? What are you aware of?

Reach your arms straight in front of your body, palms facing each other, relaxed and not rigid. With each exhale, extend your awareness out of your fingertips, imagining awareness traveling beyond your body into the open space in front of you. Relax your posture and allow your mind to rest, feeling and sensing the space in front of you. Bring in an awareness of the back of your body.

You can now return to the original posture, arms to the sides, palms down. Begin to move your arms along the horizontal plane, breathing your awareness out through the fingertips, feeling your energetic extension through the entire 360-degree circumference of your body. When you feel finished, add in the vertical plane, extending your arms above your head. Feel the breath—and your awareness—exit your fingertips toward the sky. Do this with the ground as well.

With each inhale, feel your center charging with breath, and with each exhale extend your breath through all of the physical planes into the space around you. Experience embodied awareness expanding. Then let go of the technique, relax your arms and your awareness, and simply notice any shift in your perception.

MULTIDIMENSIONAL CAPACITY

Psychedelic therapists play a crucial role in containing their clients' experience. This requires an ethical commitment to therapeutic boundaries (see Chapter 2) and familiarity with possible adverse events (see Chapter 5). In addition, we need to have a sense of multidimensionality, allowing our awareness to be grounded and sensitively attuned.

Psychedelics connect us to realms of the numinous, and initiate nonlinear psychological processing. This multidimensional state of being is dynamic and ever changing. It can include contradictory messages, symbols, and visions, challenging the solidity of our ordinary experience. To hold and integrate the paradoxical qualities of nonordinary states requires multidimensional presence.

Therapists must be comfortable with nonduality and able to hold ambiguous, conflicting truths. We must also be able to adapt quickly to sudden shifts in the client's journey. In one moment, the client may be in the throes of an emotional release, leaning into our support—in the next, experiencing a state of union with the divine—and then, suddenly, try to leave the premises, requiring us to set an unwavering boundary. There's simply no predicting when these shifts will happen. The key is to have confidence that we can hold the client's experience in all its multiplicity. We practice an engaged kind of waiting, staying close to our own internal experience and allowing our interactions with the client to emerge organically. In doing so, we implicitly welcome the entirety of their being, however it may show up in the session.

As we prepare for multidimensionality, it can be valuable to make sure that we therapists feel supported too. One of the things you can do is call upon allies, nonphysical beings that can accompany you as you hold space for others. For instance, you could visualize a supportive presence drawing close and standing with or behind you. This could be an ancestor, teacher, or mentor (living or deceased). Or this could be an animal, or any other transpersonal entity. Whether you believe these presences are truly there in an energetic sense—or simply imagined—this visualization will change your state of being. Don't struggle too hard to get it "right," trusting what comes and reminding yourself that it's about *being*, not *doing*.

CORE COMPETENCIES OF THE PSYCHEDELIC THERAPIST

Many schools of psychedelic therapy list the fundamental values and practices necessary for this work. For instance, Phelps (2017) catalogued core competencies for psychedelic therapists, and MAPS did the same in its manual for MDMA-AT (Mithoefer, 2016). We emphasize four competencies that we consider indispensable: embodied presence, grounded compassion, awareness of the relational field, and holding space for the inner healer.

We begin by entering a state of *embodied presence*. The more the therapist can ground themselves in their own somatic awareness, the more permission the client will feel to fully inhabit and express their state of being. Remember, our goal is to be attuned to what occurs, without judgment or agenda, embracing that what is happening *just is*. In this state, the therapist's body, breath, heart, and mind can be aligned, initiating receptivity and curiosity. This will be palpable to the client. Once established, embodied presence allows us to enter a state of engaged waiting, in which we neither pull away nor hurry the process.

The receptivity of embodied presence naturally gives rise to *grounded compassion*—a heart-centered attunement with the client, empathy in action, with a fundamentally open and nonjudgmental attitude. This requires engaged listening—beneath and beyond words—for deeper meanings. The therapist is relaxed. They ask questions, exploring without prying. We genuinely delight in the client's accomplishments, conveying our appreciation for them.

Grounded compassion awakens our *awareness of the relational field* between therapist and client. We join with the client and allow ourselves to be moved by their process, feeling tender in their moments of suffering and rejoicing in their moments of joy or insight, celebrating their growth and change.

The relationship between client and therapist is a sacred connection, a field of awareness that is co-created, a shared interpersonal space. It can be useful to recognize that within every pairing of individuals there is also a *third*: the energetic entity that comprises the relationship between them. This intersubjective field is ever present, and by purposefully cultivating our sensing of it we honor both interactants, as well as the third—our shared being.

Once we are nonjudgmentally present, with an awareness of the relational field, *holding space for the inner healer* simply happens on its own. The therapist rests in open awareness, watching and listening with steadiness. Within this open space, the client can move through the trials of the journey without being interrupted, trusting their own inner healing intelligence to show them the way. Holding space, when done with skill, activates latent resources in the client's psyche. The therapist waits, with their full attention on whatever emerges. No agenda, no plan, no expectation. We simply witness and receive.

The clinician's role is to trust, recognizing that the journeyer has the capacity to transform trauma and distress—if given the right conditions (Mithoefer, 2016). The principle of inner healing intelligence holds that all living systems have a self-correcting directive and an innate drive to reestablish equilibrium (Vaid & Walker, 2022). Hakomi refers to this way of holding the process as organicity, recognizing a self-organizing tendency within the psyche (Johanson, 2015; Kurtz, 2015). Levine (1997) describes how the SE methodology allows people to "begin to recognize the ways in which [one's] body attempts to heal itself" and helps the practitioner learn to "support rather than impede this innate capacity for healing" (p. 12). This is intrinsic in each of us, inner rhythms and unconscious processes moving toward wholeness. The therapist's presence supports the client to trust in their evolving process.

Contemplative practice can be a tremendous aid to the process of holding space for the inner healing intelligence, particularly systems of meditation emphasizing nondual awareness (such as *mahamudra* and *dzogchen*). Another powerful way to build our capacity for holding space is by tuning into the felt sense.

Try This: Tuning Into the Felt Sense

- Let your mind settle, drawing a few slow, even breaths into the lower belly.
- Now picture your client and the work ahead, holding them in your awareness.
- Notice what feelings arise as you see your client in your mind's eye. Would you describe this felt experience as excitement? Curiosity? Anxiety? Dread?

- What do you notice in your body as you focus on your client? Does the quality of your breathing change? Do you feel tension? Spaciousness? Heat? Pressure?
- Pay close attention and notice whatever comes up. Tune into the sensations, emotions, and images. Let go of any interpretations.
- What is the felt sense revealing to you about this client and your orientation to them?

THE SACREDNESS OF HOLDING SPACE

Simply holding space is a sacred activity, requiring that we not be distracted. We empty ourselves of extraneous concerns. This creates psychospiritual receptivity, borne of our own curiosity about how the cosmos expresses itself through this unique individual.

In the Lakota tradition it is said that the medicine person must be a *hollow bone*. Emptying allows the healer to become a channel for the spirits, essences, and energies that accomplish the healing. The efficacy of the treatment depends upon the openness of the healer, whether their body and mind are clear enough to be a conduit for transpersonal allies. Regardless of our beliefs, this principle is instructive for psychedelic-assisted therapy. The therapist needs to bring less of their *small self* to the session, less ego striving, less conditioned awareness.

A similar principle is found in some meditative traditions. *Pure awareness*, in these practices, describes cognition freed from content, a wordless attention that enables participation in the here and now. In Taoism, a state called *wu wei* (sometimes translated as "the action of nonaction") is sometimes achieved by contemplatives or martial artists. *Wu wei* signifies an effective but "effortless" performance of one's duties. When awareness is clarified, we may find ourselves less interested in prefiguring outcomes, instead speaking and behaving without a preordained goal. In these moments, we may find our action effortlessly aligned with the rhythms and directionality of our deepest nature.

The therapist rests in open space, allowing the client to move through challenges without being interrupted. This person is potentially meeting with transpersonal beings or energies, angels or demons, and we need to take care not to clutter that space with interventions. This is profoundly different from normal psychotherapy, and differs markedly from most interactions one has in life. As the client is called to trust their own inner healer, we nonverbally model faith in the process.

This kind of waiting is both anticipatory and relaxed, active and allowing. Often, therapists either relax too much, becoming subtly disengaged, or they become overly attached to the process unfolding before them, trying to direct it toward preordained ends.

Try This: Meet Your Compassionate Heart

This can be a helpful practice when you feel resistance or blockage toward your client. Imagine a recent client who you want to feel more compassion toward. Notice where and how your experience is blocked or stuck. How does this show up? Somatically or mentally? Do you feel a judgment arise? Do you want to dismiss their story? Do you feel burdened or triggered by them? Notice your somatic response to this client. You can write down a couple of words or say them out loud. Let go of any judgment or dismissive feelings. Now, intentionally, remember the kind of suffering behind their story. What do you imagine they feel when they are alone or faced with their situation? How did they arrive in this place of shame or guilt? What do you imagine their inner world feels like? Place your hand on your heart center and make a well-intentioned, heartful wish to alleviate their suffering. Wish them genuine ease from their pain. For example, you can say, "I wish you relief and ease from your pain." You can say this a few times until you feel a softening inside. Then, follow up by telling yourself, "Your pain is not my pain." Say this a few times until you feel something change inside. This could be a somatic shift, leading to new feelings about that client. What happens inside of you?

BECOMING TRAUMA INFORMED

Being knowledgeable about trauma, and how trauma symptoms manifest in the body, is an essential skill set. The capacity to read somatic markers is key for determining which (if any) interventions to use.

However, an awareness of trauma cuts both ways. As we develop our ability to hold space, we discover that self-regulation and managing our own triggers are crucial. In challenging sessions—for example, when a client's psyche is processing trauma, panic, or recounting horrific events—the therapist may become stressed. When this occurs—and it *will* occur—there can be a tendency to off-load our own distress by diving headlong into the client's process. Feeling helpless and wanting to be useful, the therapist intervenes. While sometimes necessary, often this only exacerbates the client's distress. Many therapeutic ruptures occur when the therapist is stressed and attempting to regulate their own nervous system by intervening, while *they* are supposed to be holding space for the *other* person. Being trauma informed is not just about the client's trauma but understanding one's own, and how it impacts the work.

This is another instance when nondual awareness comes to our aid. As we steady ourselves in our multidimensional seat, we can attend to our own distress and the client's distress simultaneously. In fact, sometimes when we focus on regulating our own system in these frightening moments—perhaps by feeling our feet on the floor and breathing into the lower belly, or by orienting to what's inside the room—we end up helping the client deactivate. We provide them with a steady nervous system to attune with, an opportunity for coregulation that positively impacts both people. To do this effectively, though, requires maintaining awareness of both ourselves and the other person. We have to be able to rub our belly while patting our head, so to speak. It is advanced work that necessitates training the mind through awareness practices, such as meditation or nature connection.

Try This: The Therapist's Intention

Many psychedelic preparation protocols involve intentions, but this is usually just for the journeyer. We think it can be important for the practitioner to develop an intention as well. Whether this is general (related to the helper's practice overall) or more specific (a goal for supporting a particular client), having a clear intention is helpful. Take time with the following invitations, curiously attending to your embodied experience as you explore what arises in your mind:

- What is it that you want to achieve?
- What beings or entities can you call upon for support?
- How can you best be a servant of the medicine?
- What qualities do you possess that will help you in this?
- What characteristics of yours might get in the way?

DEVELOPING MULTIDIMENSIONAL CAPACITY

Indigenous medicine traditions train practitioners over the course of years—or even decades—in long apprenticeships with master healers. These apprenticeships are designed to train the person from the inside out. In our medicalized Western model of therapy, we often train from the outside in, focusing on techniques and theories that lack any dimension of interiority. Because internal experience is so central to psychedelic work, it is essential that Western psychedelic therapists cultivate awareness of our own inner landscape. This means committing to continuous practice and education, a journey of discovery and learning that never ends.

We must develop awareness of our inner state, consciously attending to this ever-shifting display of internal experiences. Meditation, yoga, dance and/or movement practices, tai chi or qigong, martial arts, herbal medicine, and earth-based practices are all valid forms of inner-state training, as are countless others. Learning to live from "the gut," from a somatically open place, will become second nature if we commit ourselves to this type of inner training. When we learn to marry our perceptions to somatic responses, or *see* from the *soma*, we can more easily notice our own biases and our own triggers. We can then work with these energies to dissipate unnecessary charge, finding ways to interact with others that are more settled and curious. By developing our multidimensional capacity we become more receptive, more able to meet life on *its* terms rather than our own. It is a strange paradox that by coming very, very close to our own experience we end up making more space for everyone else. Be curious, and remain open to learning from life's mysteries.

Try This: Somatic Opening

To see from the soma means learning to be present to our inner state without judgment, simply noticing what arises. We are learning to observe what is happening inside, as a form of gathering information, resisting the impulse to immediately interpret or create meaning. This takes practice, but once we learn to be with our own soma while we guide, we realize how indispensable this is.

The practice below is a skillful way to train your multidimensional capacity. We encourage you to do it often. Read over the instructions first, perhaps memorizing the basic steps, and reviewing as necessary as you follow the protocol.

1. Take a comfortable position: sitting, lying down, or standing. Find a posture that relaxes you but does not make you sleepy.
2. Set a timer for 15 minutes.
3. Now, settle into your posture and observe your state of being. Slowly sweep your attention from your head to your feet, noticing whatever is happening inside.
4. Place one hand on your belly and the other on your chest. Become curious about the specific way your breath is moving your body right now.
5. Wait until something inside changes—perhaps a deeper, more spontaneous breath, or a release of tension. The specifics aren't important, just look for anything new arising that captures your attention. Try not to label it or tell yourself a story about what it means.
6. If your attention becomes fixed on this novel occurrence, soften it a bit.
7. Now expand your focus to include your entire body. You aren't scanning, or looking for anything in particular—it's a process of engaged waiting for anything to shift, to open.
8. Where do you notice these openings? Your foot? Your chest? What are their qualities? Do you feel heaviness?

Spaciousness? Heat? Brilliance? These may be subtle at first.
9. Let your attention rest on your breath for a moment. Then once again, widen your inner focus, listen, and receive. Let yourself be with whatever comes up, without any reactivity, labeling, or judgment.
10. If thoughts arise, let them drift away like clouds, and return to sensation.
11. When the timer goes off at 15 minutes, relax your focus, let go of the technique, open your eyes, and notice the quality of your awareness in this moment.
12. Reflect on these questions in writing:
    - How am I feeling in this moment?
    - How am I receiving my body?
    - Where in my body are there somatic openings?
    - What is my body trying to communicate to me right now?

CONCLUSION

Preparation is a critical component of psychedelic therapy, for the therapist as well as the client. The guide's internal state sets the baseline for the journeyer's experience, and the quality of the guide's attention directly impacts the character of the journey.

A primary goal of the preparation phase is to establish sufficient safety for the client, allowing them to trust, let go, and open to the psychedelic experience. This sense of safety is first established unconsciously through neuroception. The therapist will be nonverbally communicating safety cues to the client through their somatic set.

Because the somatic set of the therapist can have such outsized influence on the client's experience, it is crucial that therapists settle their own nervous system. This implicitly signals trust to the client, and can help contain the intensity of the medicine session. Therapists must cultivate habits and practices that allow them to be attentive and present, both to their own experience and to the client's. They must also establish comfort with ambiguity and nonduality as they hold space for the client. Psychedelic journeys are multidimensional, and the person holding space must be as well.

We turn our attention now to the preparation session, as the client makes ready for their journey. The next chapter explores in detail the myriad ways we can collaborate with clients to build a safe container for the psychedelic experience.

CHAPTER 7

Preparing the Client

They are powerful tools and, like any tool, they can be used skillfully, ineptly, or destructively. The result will be critically dependent on the set and setting.
—STANISLAV GROF

The most important step in any journey is the first. Adequate preparation will make or break any adventure, steadying us in moments of unforeseen adversity. It's like backpacking. Forget to bring that crucial piece of gear—or fail to research the climate and terrain of the place you'll be visiting—and you could end up suffering rather than connecting with nature and being rejuvenated. Preparing for the psychedelic experience is no different. In this chapter, we focus on the importance of the preparation stage in the three-part sequence outlined in the Introduction (preparation, journey, integration).

SCREENING AND INTAKE

Before preparing clients for psychedelic-assisted therapy we want to make sure they are properly screened. As stated in the Introduction, not everyone will benefit from psychedelic therapy, and there are possible contraindications for this treatment. In fact, psychedelic researchers often disqualify people from studies who have a family history of psychosis, bipolar I disorder, or extreme emotional instability. The psychedelic therapist must carefully consider whether a particular person will profit from taking these powerful drugs at this particular time.

Psychedelics are generally considered very safe. There is no known lethal dose of a substance like LSD, and even accidental overdoses hundreds of times the usual amount have not been fatal. For most people, enduring negative effects are rare. Again, however, people with a history of schizophrenia (or who have first-order family members with such a history) could have a psychotic break after a psychedelic experience. Those diagnosed with bipolar I may suffer a manic episode after a journey. It's safer for individuals with a history of mental breakdown to explore gentle somatic approaches rather than psychedelics.

Various hallucinogens, as well as MDMA (a methamphetamine), exert strong effects on the cardiovascular system—people with high blood pressure or cardiovascular issues should be carefully screened. Diabetes, which can involve occult cardiovascular disease, is another potential red flag for the therapist. A history of stroke should similarly raise alarms, as well as any disease involving the liver or kidneys, since the body must be able to eliminate these substances after a session. Because psychedelics sometimes create nausea and vomiting, someone with an esophageal fissure or gastric ulcers could be negatively affected. Suggesting a checkup prior to the journey is a good idea. The consent form(s) should require the client to state whether they have had such a checkup, or at least that they have no medical condition of which they are aware that would make psychedelic therapy a medical or psychological risk.

A client might also speak with their primary care doctor or other medical professionals about psychedelic-assisted therapy. For instance, they can ask if there are any contraindications in their health profile. They can introduce the topic by first emphasizing the proven efficacy of these treatments, describing how they want the *right to try* psychedelics to treat their bodily or psychological complaints. Some physicians and psychiatrists are willing to consult with current patients "off chart," while others will choose not to speak about these matters—but it's not illegal to ask. Some doctors now even advertise checkups for psychedelic therapy candidates.

In the preparation stage, the therapist must assess the person's overall physiological health and psychological stability. Although psychedelic-assisted therapy is likely to be beneficial in the long term, it can be acutely destabilizing in the short term. A degree of resilience and good *ego strength*—the ability to withstand challenges to one's psychic structure—are critical.

If the person has disordered eating, particularly if this involves purging, psychedelics might not be the treatment of choice. Suicidality is also something the therapist should carefully consider. Past suicidal ideation would not be a rule out for many psychedelic therapists. If the person is currently suicidal, however, it's best to do stabilizing work until the crisis has passed.

Clients with borderline personality disorder (BPD) may have challenges integrating the psychedelic experience. The therapist could suggest other approaches first, such as dialectical behavior therapy or somatic work. While the classic psychedelics could prove troublesome for clients with BPD, some researchers speculate that MDMA-AT may have the potential to improve treatment outcomes for individuals with BPD (Traynor et al., 2022).

Another consideration is dissociation. Some people tend to leave their bodies, or have an eerie sense that things are unreal. Clients prone to dissociate in response to intense experiences—a common reaction to unhealed trauma—may struggle to benefit from psychedelic experiences. As with other indications above, somatic work to address dysregulation in the nervous system would be more beneficial—and this could prepare the person for a later foray into psychedelic states.

One important element of preparation is communicating how hard psychedelic journeys are. While some lucky people experience uninterrupted cosmic bliss during their expanded state, most journeys include phases of pain and fear, where we come face-to-face with our trauma, our habitual patterns, and our shame and grief. We might feel paranoia, exaltation, emptiness, and relaxation, all in the same session.

To assess who is a good candidate during the preparation stage, the therapist should emphasize how challenging journeys can be and see how this is received. People might gravitate toward psychedelics because they habitually crave intensity. Getting repetitively overstimulated may not be helpful, though, and a journey could reinforce patterns of *sensation seeking*—being repetitively drawn to risky, high-intensity activities—that keep them overwhelmed in life.

Others may be drawn to psychedelics because they've heard these are miracle drugs that will magically resolve their trauma. They may want to use psychedelics as a way to spiritually bypass their psychological issues. Clients should be informed that what is most likely to occur in their journey is an alternation between pleasure and pain, ease and challenge—and, in fact, this oscillation is part of the psychedelic experience's transformative power. However, for this to be effective the person must be in a state of receptivity, of nonresistance. We cultivate this attitude in the preparation stage.

The therapist should let clients know that one journey is usually not enough. People undergoing psychedelic therapy often find it necessary to do a series of journeys to make substantive progress toward their therapeutic goals. Many among the psychedelically curious expect the experience to be a "one and done," a psychic surgery that will remove all of their unmetabolized distress. Unfortunately, there is little evidence to support this belief. Very few of the research studies proving psilocybin is an effective treatment for depression (e.g., Davis et al., 2021)—or MDMA is an effective treatment for PTSD (e.g., Mitchell et al., 2023)—were one-session protocols. This work often necessitates a period of regular exposure to expanded states (though we do recommend taking significant breaks between journeys, at least at first).

In the preparation stage, therapists collect information from prospective journeyers. Each practitioner has a different approach to this intake process. Some use complicated, multipage forms, asking clients for extensive details on their personal history. For some clients, this may constitute an invitation to ruminate, alone, on the unfortunate circumstances of their lives. Clients with a significant trauma history, or who have experienced abuse from caregivers, may have a hard time filling out these forms at home. We should be careful to avoid overwhelm, and it may be better to interview such clients face-to-face. Part of creating the right mental set for effective therapy is learning about a person's history without awakening the demons of their past. However we decide to conduct the intake, some basic biographical information should be collected, as this prepares the therapist for the themes and emotional content that could arise in the journey. This could include details about their family of origin, trauma history, list of personal resources, and a description of current relationships that are supportive and safe.

Drug Interactions

The therapist must know which medications the client takes, or has taken in the past, as these can significantly impact the way psychedelics affect the brain. The classic psychedelics work primarily through the 5-HT2A receptors ("5-HT" being the technical term for the neurotransmitter serotonin). Therefore, psychiatric medications targeting the serotonin system (including the popular SSRIs [*selective serotonin reuptake inhibitors*], such as Prozac) can interfere with the effect of psychedelics.

Most longtime users of SSRIs report that their medication causes a "blunting" of the psychedelic state. Heavy doses of psychedelics often have diminished subjective effects for these individuals. For this reason, psychedelic therapists in the underground encourage clients to taper off their SSRIs before the dosing session. Besides eliminating the blunting effect, the client's willingness to taper off their meds signifies their commitment to the journey, and is an important aspect of preparing to let go and open.

Of course, it is outside any psychotherapist's scope of practice to give medical advice or suggest ignoring a prescriber's protocol. In Oregon, where clinical use of psilocybin is legal, licensed psilocybin facilitators are similarly prevented from advising clients on their medication regimen. Whether the guide or therapist suggests anything to the client about the use of SSRIs, it is still important to know what medications they take, as this aids the selection of an appropriate dose of psychedelic medicine.

A note of caution: When someone takes a serotonergic psychedelic while already on a serotonin reuptake inhibitor, there is a small but nontrivial risk of developing *serotonin syndrome*: a potentially fatal physiological emergency when circulating serotonin levels become too high. (This is particularly true when a monoamine oxidase inhibitor [MAOI] is involved in the psychedelic preparation, as it is in the ayahuasca brew.)

Some physicians (including naturopathic doctors) are knowledgeable about the interaction of psychedelics with various psychiatric drugs, and the therapist can refer clients to these practitioners prior to the dosing session.

Adverse physiological reactions of various kinds can occur on psychedelics. Therefore, therapists should know the location of the nearest emergency room and make a hospital transport plan. Again, as with all possible adverse effects and consequences, the client should consent to this plan in writing during the preparation stage. Though this has only very, very rarely been needed, it is important to have contingencies in place.

Confidentiality and Fee Structure

Discussing confidentiality during the intake process is important. The therapist should let the client know how they plan to safeguard their personal information, and go over any policies around recordkeeping. The goal of the preparation session is to make all involved feel reasonably comfortable before the journey. The therapist shows the journeyer that there is a container for the session, an energetic boundary to protect the experience. The therapist should also clarify what information about their practice they are comfortable with the client sharing. Owing to the legal status of some psychedelics, the therapist may ask that their identity be kept secret until they give explicit permission to be named.

We should be transparent about our fee structure from the start, making sure there will be no surprises regarding payment for our services. Many psychedelic therapists offer a set fee for the entire package of preparation session(s), dosing session, and integration session(s), while others may charge an hourly rate. Some therapists may opt to provide only a piece of this package to a particular client, such as integration sessions for a journey the client did with a different guide. Regardless, the client should be informed in writing of the total cost, as well as when and how payment is to be provided. The last thing we want is for the therapeutic efficacy of the work to be derailed by the client's surprise at the fee—or worse, for the client to leave the session feeling commercially exploited by the therapist.

THE PREPARATION SESSION

Spirituality

In the preparation stage, we explore the client's spiritual beliefs. Transpersonal or transcendent elements are consistent features of the psychedelic experience. As mentioned, research suggests that journeys containing a *mystical-type experience* result in greater therapeutic gains (Griffiths et al., 2008, 2016). Unfortunately, some popular guidebooks for psychedelic therapy seem to suggest there is a preferred metaphysical orientation, with guided meditations and rituals that prescribe a specific approach to spirituality. We instead suggest that any spiritual aspects should be tailored to the journeyer, arising out of their personal relationship with spirituality or divinity. You might even collaborate with the client to design a ritual beginning the journey, one that is relevant to their spiritual practice and belief system. As therapists, we must be careful that our own spiritual bias doesn't creep in, and recognize the value of each journeyer's unique way of connecting—or not connecting—with what lies beyond. We should also be open to surprises. Journeyers may report powerful encounters with deities outside their faith tradition, and even atheists sometimes find themselves connecting with energies that transcend their understanding.

Preparation and the Body

Engaging the body is helpful in the preparation stage. Somatic therapies and psychedelic experiences share key features: bottom-up processing, letting go, and accepting novel insights as they emerge from the deepest strata of the psyche. To engage clients somatically is to initiate them into mystery, teaching them how to listen to the wordless language of the body. This can be thought of as a "practice lap" for the psychedelic experience. Therapists should encourage their clients to track sensations, scanning their bodies to learn what the unconscious is sharing with them (as mentioned, the technical term for this inner sensing is "interoception"). The therapist should also pay attention to the client's bodily posture, gestural communication, facial expressions, and other cues, reflecting back to the client the *body narrative* being expressed in each moment. A greater understanding of what's happening below the threshold of awareness will serve the client when they are in an expanded state. Preparatory sessions with a qualified somatic therapist—whether the psychedelic therapist themselves or via a referral to a different practitioner—will make the journey far more fruitful.

Preparatory sessions should include practices for grounding and stabilizing. Using breath and body awareness to come back to one's center may come in handy as the psychedelic drug sets in, and the journeyer should be given tools to work with high-intensity states. These aren't offered to give our clients more control over their experience but rather as ways for the client to ground themselves and be open to whatever unfolds. Having taught these techniques in advance, the therapist can then offer reminders of these practices—or even guide the client through them—if things become overly intense in the medicine session.

Intentions

Another key aspect of preparation involves the client's intention for the journey. The question of forming intentions for psychedelic therapy is hotly debated within the field. The psychedelic pioneer Ralph Metzner (2015) believed intentions to be crucial, and strongly suggested his clients form clear intentions prior to the experience. Other guides suggest that intentions can cloud a person's mental space, narrowing attention in a way that constrains the possibilities inherent in the journey.

Our perspective is that intentions are helpful, provided they are *lightly held* and *easily relinquished*. Sometimes what comes to pass has little to do with the intention. However, being clear about our aims for the work may provide some structural scaffolding for the process. The therapist may remind the journeyer of their intention at some point in the journey, if the theme doesn't arise organically. Doing this can also be a useful way to help the journeyer focus and recenter if their cognition becomes scattered or confused. Interoception should be woven into the crafting of intention, tracking the body's response to statements about what the conscious mind hopes might happen. Clients may discover that the body has different intentions than the mind.

Part of this relates to expectations. Clients may be experienced with psychedelics, either therapeutically or recreationally, but it's important for them to know that each journey is unique. A psychedelic experience with a group of friends at a festival may prove starkly different from an inwardly focused psychedelic journey with guidance and support. Similarly, psychedelics won't work the same for everyone. Clients may have heard accounts of miraculous experiences from friends or in the media, but any attempt to make their journey conform to what they're expecting could interfere with their own unique process.

Resistance Is Futile

What is paramount in preparing for a journey is to, as Frank Herbert (2003) wrote in *Dune*, "Be prepared to appreciate what you meet" (p. 322). Unexpected happenings should be expected: the irruption of memories, often with a vividness and emotional weight that takes the journeyer by force; the emergence of insights, crushing or liberating or filled with spiritual import; experiences in the body, such as involuntary movement patterns or what is sometimes called *discharge*—shaking or trembling; or even, at higher doses, the temporary dissolution of one's very self.

If there's one universal principle among the myriad expressions of the psychedelic journey, it's that we must be receptive to what transpires. Or, as the Borg (in *Star Trek*) put it, "Resistance is futile." That is to say, if the journeyer tries to control the process, it will almost always go awry, and their primary task is to—as psychedelic researchers at Johns Hopkins put it—"TLO: Trust, Let go, and be Open" (Richards, 2015, p. 35). Clients should be encouraged to turn toward the experience, interacting with the play of images, emotions, sensations, and thoughts, led by nothing other than curiosity, even when things are scary . . . or perhaps, *especially* when things are scary. Let them know that if a monster shows up in the journey, they can meet it with curiosity, allowing themselves to befriend even those demons that seem tailor-made to drive them into a panic. And if bliss shows up, let them know that they can relax and enjoy it, not squelching transcendent experiences with doubt or second-guessing.

Risks and Complications

The preparation session should involve informing journeyers about the risks involved in psychedelic therapy. In the current wave of enthusiasm for this work, real concerns are sometimes swept away with the cavalier confidence of the zealous. While ongoing psychiatric distress after a journey is rare, it does happen, especially for the aforementioned vulnerable people (who should be screened out). These experiences can dramatically alter one's perspective on life, leading people to question their careers, marriages, and other life circumstances.

We believe it's worth highlighting these realities, not to kindle fear or reactivity but to deepen acceptance of change. When someone takes a psychedelic, there is a turning point from which they may never return, at least not in the same condition. While most people feel normal within hours after the drug wears off—and are often dismayed at the resurgence of their accustomed neurotic fixations and limitations—it is possible that they will emerge transformed into a new way of being: truer, more open, and free. To protect and reinforce these delicate shifts of consciousness, the therapist can invite the client to share the experience only with their most trusted people, those who are likely to affirm its value and to help them integrate it into their life.

The underground therapist Leo Zeff, profiled in the book *The Secret Chief Revealed* (Stolaroff, 2004), employed a metaphor that many journeyers relate to: the "castle analogy." Normally the subconscious is kept behind a locked door, a fortified entrance allowing only occasional glimpses into the castle. When under the influence of a psychedelic, however, the gate opens and we can explore the castle for a time. We can traverse different floors, different rooms, perhaps even delve into the dank basement to see what's living down there. Some of what we find might be frightening, but the openness of the castle is a golden opportunity. Eventually we will leave and the gate will close again, but we will never forget all that we encountered in that fortress, even when we are beyond its walls. Sharing analogies such as this can be helpful in preparation sessions, especially for first-time users.

Another suggestion of Zeff's, part of creating a strong container for the work, is to set *ground rules* (Stolaroff, 2004). We might tell clients that it's okay to experience whatever comes up without judgment or resistance, but we *will not* allow certain things to occur. These could include physically harming the therapist, physically harming themselves, leaving the property while under the influence, making phone calls or sending texts under the influence, any form of sexual contact between therapist and journeyer, and so on.

During preparation, Zeff would tell his clients something like "You need to agree that in your journey, if I tell you to do something—or to stop doing something—you will" (Stolaroff, 2004). While this kind of unilateral authority may be hard for some clients to stomach, it is useful to get consent in advance that they will fully let the therapist guide them. Whatever agreement is made between therapist and client about this, it should be documented in writing. Paranoia comes up in journeys, but can be mitigated by the remembrance that the guide was once seen as trustworthy enough to have been given a promise of compliance. If a person gets stuck in an overwhelming emotional experience, and convinced that some kind of destructive behavior is necessary, it can help them to realize that the guide is sober and able to more accurately assess the implications.

They may be convinced they need to flee, but we mustn't let this happen. As the American Psychedelic Practitioners Association (APPA; 2023) states, "patients . . . may withdraw their consent to treatment at any time, [but] such withdrawal does not supersede the need to remain onsite until it is safe for them to leave" (p. 17).

We should also inform clients that it is not unusual for *trans-*

ference to occur in the journey. This psychoanalytic term describes a tendency to relate with people in the here and now as if they are powerful figures from the past, such as caregivers. In other words, they *transfer* a relationship with someone else onto the relationship they have with the therapist. The journeyer may behave toward the therapist in a particular way that recalls this past relationship, or could even hallucinate that the therapist has become this person. Therapists should recognize and name these projections, differentiating ourselves from the projected person, even asking what comes up in the journeyer's body as these projections are identified and explored.

We want to make sure that our alliance with the journeyer remains intact throughout the process. Of course, things do come up and there can be ruptures in rapport, but if the client comes to mistrust the therapist and gets stuck in a defensive interpersonal posture, it can hinder the healing potential of the journey.

We should remember that not every practitioner is the right fit for each client. We should not rush prospective journeyers, encouraging them to take their time and assess whether they truly feel ready—and if they're sure we're the right person for them. In the past, we've suggested to potential clients that they interview other therapists and/or guides, letting them know it's wise to "shop around" before selecting the person they will grant this sacred role. They can ask about the person's training and experience, and ask themselves: "Will I feel relatively comfortable relinquishing control with this person holding the safety net?"

PHYSICAL TOUCH AND THE PHYSICAL SPACE

One tool the therapist can use to help stabilize the journeyer—as well as kindle warm feelings of connection—is physical contact. Healthy touch maintains appropriate boundaries and respects the bodily autonomy of the client, while it provides greater containment and energetic support. Touch could look like holding the client's hand, offering them a shoulder to cry on, or some other kind of physical contact. It often helps clients to ground into embodied experience when someone touches them, particularly if the journey becomes challenging. After all, touch is our first language, the language of the body.

Sometimes clients will have a hard time forming words, and may struggle to understand us. In these moments, touch may be our main—or only—intervention. We introduce the possibility of touch in the preparation session, determining whether contact is desired and how best to implement it in the journey (see Chapter 10 for more information on touch).

If possible, the client should see the room where their journey will occur. This allows them to acclimate to the setting while in normal, waking consciousness. The therapist can inquire with the client how to make the space feel more like home to them. Many psychedelic therapists have an altar in their treatment room, and will invite clients to bring items to place upon it, infusing the space with the client's own energies and intent. The therapist should clarify who will be there during the journey, orienting the client to the presence of any others on the premises. The therapist should also inform the client that they will take bathroom breaks, snack breaks, or other forms of self-care.

TYPES OF MEDICINE

Another question that will need to be raised in the preparation stage regards the choice of medicine. At the time of this writing, the only classic psychedelic my [Joshua] home state of Oregon legally allows is psilocybin, which must be administered in a licensed service center and overseen by a licensed facilitator.

Knowing that the rescheduling of many of these medicines is on the horizon, and that some journeyers will be motivated to seek out psychedelic medicines before they're decriminalized, we treat this issue in an open-ended way.

The "classic psychedelics" include LSD, psilocybin, mescaline, and dimethyltryptamine (DMT). A host of other analogues and "designer drugs" have sprung up in recent decades, some of which are also 5-HT2A receptor agonists, and some of which exert psychedelic effects through different neurological processes. Each of these drugs has a different time course, with differing psychological effects and somatic signatures. Some theorists, such as William Richards (2015), suggest that each of the various psychedelics open pathways to a limitless variety of transformative states (a "skeleton key"), while others differentiate the classics from one another in terms of their effects, utilizing different medicines at different points to achieve different outcomes. While all of these drugs alter aspects of basic functioning (visual and auditory effects, time perception, etc.), they do so in somewhat characteristic ways. We describe some commonly held ideas about them below, but these descriptions are very general. Each one will impact different people in different ways:

> Psilocybin: The various psilocybin-containing "magic mushrooms" (which additionally contain other psychoactive compounds) have been transforming human consciousness for millennia. There is also chemically synthesized psilocybin, a tryptamine, which has been utilized in many research studies. This compound ushers in a 4- to 6-hour altered state in which distorted sensory perceptions, time dilation, and novel insights can occur. A common therapeutic dose is 2.0–3.5 grams of dried mushroom, roughly equivalent to 20–35 milligrams of

synthesized psilocybin (dried mushrooms vary enormously in their psilocybin content, and this conversion is offered as only the roughest approximation).

LSD: First synthesized in 1938, the lysergamide *lysergic acid diethylamide* has a storied history in Western culture. It is less commonly employed in psychedelic therapy nowadays, but was rigorously studied in the 1950s and 1960s. LSD intoxication lasts 8–10 hours. While many of its acute effects are similar to psilocybin, it is often reported to elicit less emotional volatility and greater cognitive clarity. An extraordinarily powerful compound, a common therapeutic dose is 100–250 *micro*grams.

Mescaline: A phenethylamine, mescaline is found in peyote, San Pedro, Peruvian torch, and other cacti. Like psilocybe mushrooms, it has evidence of human use going back thousands of years. Western scientists first identified the compound in 1897. It's a longer-acting material, often lasting 10–12 hours. Its effects are sometimes described as subtler and gentler than other psychedelics, with vivid colors and a sense of directly perceiving one's surroundings without mental filters. A common therapeutic dose is 200–400 milligrams.

DMT: *N,N-dimethyltryptamine* and its close cousin *5-methoxy-N,N-dimethyltryptamine* (5-MeO-DMT), though distinct in certain ways, are both shorter acting than the other psychedelics, with more distorting effects on consciousness. The DMT-containing brew ayahuasca, consumed in various South American indigenous cultures, is ceremonially used in groups and less often in one-on-one psychedelic therapy contexts. DMT can also be smoked, vaped, or insufflated (snorted through nasal passages). Taken orally, it will not be psychoactive unless administered with a monoamine oxidase (MAO) inhibitor, as it is in the ayahuasca recipe. 5-MeO-DMT is found in certain plants, as well as the skin excretions of some toad species. What all DMTs seem to share is the ability to rapidly induce a powerfully altered state, one in which ineffable experiences are common. People may find themselves traveling to other realms, meeting sentient entities, and transcending conventional reality. The DMTs come on fast, take people far, and then return them quickly. Vaporized N,N-DMT lasts less than an hour, and 5-MeO-DMT is of a similar duration. Ayahuasca is longer lasting, and ceremonies often involve repeated dosing. Given the wide array of plants and formulations to produce DMT, estimating a therapeutic dose is not possible.

As mentioned, there are many alternatives to these "classics," some of which are preferred by therapists for various reasons. The underground chemist Alexander "Sasha" Shulgin, who sampled an untold number of substances in his decades-long quest to explore psychedelic analogues, said 2C-B (*4-bromo-2,5-dimethoxyphenethylamine*) was his favorite (Morris & Smith, 2013). It was later used extensively in underground psychedelic therapy circles. Shulgin once said it was "one of the most graceful . . . compounds I have ever invented," and that "its effects are felt very much in the body, as well as in the mind" (Center for Cognitive Liberty and Ethics, 2003, para. 5).

Another medicine is ibogaine (*12-methoxyibogamine*), often employed in the treatment of addictions. This material is derived from the iboga tree (*Tabernanthe iboga*), native to central Africa. Ibogaine is said to blunt opioid withdrawal symptoms while it occasions a psychedelic experience that makes users lose interest in their addictive habit.

In addition to the various psychedelics, there are a host of other medicines that can create psychedelic-like effects and are used for their therapeutic potential. While not included in the psychedelic class of drugs, they are increasingly considered to be part of psychedelic-assisted therapy, and employed by many therapists in this field. These include:

MDMA (*methylenedioxymethamphetamine*): Originally synthesized by Merck in 1912, it wasn't until Sasha Shulgin rediscovered MDMA that it entered psychotherapeutic practice. It is a methamphetamine, but owing to its prosocial effects, its class is sometimes identified by the neologism "empathogen," as it evokes a sense of sympathy or affection for others and for oneself. Some prefer the term "entactogen," signifying a substance that helps one contact an inner self or life. In the 1970s, it was widely adopted in underground therapy circles for work with couples, as it creates greater emotional openness and a desire for intimacy. MDMA intoxication lasts 4–6 hours. Common street names are "Molly," and also "Ecstasy," because it evokes a positive mood and sensations of pleasure in the body. Physical movement (such as dancing) and tactile stimulation are often intensely pleasurable. A common therapeutic dose is 75–125 milligrams.

Ketamine: This material is also unique, as it is a dissociative anesthetic. At certain doses, though, it can induce a psychedelic-like state with intense visual imagery and a felt sense of dissolution (as a dissociative, it can disconnect journeyers from their bodies). Used in the treatment of depression, research indicates that it is effective at ameliorating depressive symptoms in the short term, but may not elicit the enduring changes in personality that psychedelics are capable of. Ketamine is the one drug on this list that has never been a Schedule I controlled substance (classified as having "no known medical use"). Therefore, therapists can legally employ ketamine, and some have suggested this is the primary reason its adoption has been so widespread. The therapeutic dose is highly contingent on the route of administration, with varying amounts needed based on whether it is injected intravenously (IV) or intramuscularly (IM), or taken orally.

Prospective journeyers thus have many options to choose from, and part of the task of preparation sessions is to select a medicine, dose, and administration method. At this time, aboveground practitioners are constrained as to which substances they can provide. Underground therapists can potentially utilize more options.

Many providers in the underground report a preference for starting with MDMA. Because it tends to be experienced as pleasurable—both in body and in mind—it can be an ideal place to begin exploring expanded states of consciousness. Progressing from MDMA to the classic psychedelics, such as psilocybin and LSD, will allow a deeper dive into the client's psychic knots and unresolved traumas. A working knowledge of the various medicine options can help journeyers make safe and informed choices.

DOSAGE

Careful dosing is a key safeguard for a beneficial experience. We recommend titrating, employing doses at the lower end of the therapeutic range first. There is an unfortunate trend in the psychedelic space to valorize heavier doses. A deep mystique surrounds the so-called heroic dose, in which people take 5 grams of dried mushroom (or an equivalent amount of other medicine). While for some this can be a liberating experience of ego dissolution, for others it's simply overwhelming and fragmenting. Five grams of dried mushroom is roughly double the usual therapeutic dose, and far higher than the doses used in any studies on psilocybin for depression. As with many things in Western culture, there is a prevalent attitude that *more is better*.

What we would say instead is that *there's nothing inherently superior about larger doses*. No evidence suggests that higher doses have more therapeutic benefit—in fact, this seems to be associated instead with an increased prevalence of adverse events (Griffiths et al., 2011). The healing is not inherent in the drugs themselves but in the journeyer's capacity to integrate the insights revealed. In fact, some seasoned psychedelic therapists maintain that the closer an altered state is to normal consciousness, the easier it is to integrate. While this may not be true in all cases, it's undeniably true that a terrifying experience of being "too high" will do nothing to help our clients.

Sometimes a supplementary dose will be employed. This is usually called a *booster*, and is given 1–2 hours after initial administration. Most of the hallmark studies in MDMA-AT for PTSD involved subjects being offered a booster, which was also commonplace in earlier work with psilocybin and other psychedelics (Thal et al., 2023). Commonly, the booster is half the initial dose (or less). Rather than making the journeyer more altered, the booster dose prolongs the time window for therapeutic work in expanded states. In other words, it's not boosting the intoxicating effects as much as it's boosting the therapeutic potential (by elongating the journey). If the journeyer tolerates coming up on the medicine well—and is not overly anxious—the therapist can offer a booster (usually prepared in advance). We inform clients about this possibility in preparation sessions, emphasizing that it will be entirely up to them if they want to take it.

LOGISTICS OF THE DOSING SESSION

Planning the day of the medicine session is an important feature of preparation. The journeyer should know of any time constraints that exist for the facility, and should schedule drop-off and pickup accordingly (they will need a designated driver). The therapist can schedule the first integration session during the preparation session, allowing the client to leave after the journey without having to wrangle their calendar. We recommend an initial integration session a day or two after the dosing session. Encourage the client to wear comfortable, loose-fitting clothing, with layers that can be donned or removed as the body goes through phases of being chilled or overly warm. They should eat lightly, or not at all, on the morning of the dosing session.

Another matter to discuss is the use of eyeshades and headphones. While not all agree, many psychedelic therapists in the Western world consider an inward journey to be optimal. An eyeshade (or sleep mask) and over-ear headphones allow the journeyer to be contained in darkness, without the sounds of the immediate environment, focusing all of their awareness internally. Of course, Indigenous groups have been successfully using psychedelics for millennia without eyeshades, and some Western therapists insist that more transformative journeys occur without music, as this allows for a more relational experience in which the journeyer is not "manipulated" by emotionally evocative music.

Whatever the format—and we think any and all can be healing, as long as the process is well contained—the journeyer should know what to expect. If music is to be played, it is ideal if it's heard simultaneously in headphones as well as speakers in the room. This allows the therapist to hear what the client is listening to—thereby tracking the process more closely—and also allows the client to stay in the stream of the music should they need to take their headphones off. If the therapist plans to use eyeshades and/or headphones, we recommend having the client practice putting them on during the preparation session, seeing what comes up as they attend to themselves with an inward focus.

MUSIC PLAYLISTS

If you plan to use music in the journey, preparation should include talking about the music and giving the journeyer a sense of what to expect. A number of publicly available playlists now exist for psychedelic therapy, some of which have been used in high-profile psychedelic research trials. The genres range from Western classical music to ambient and new age music, world music, as well as modern "postrock" or indie music. A common thread with all of these is that the songs are nearly always instrumental—or at least do not feature lyrics in a language the client speaks. Easily understood lyrics tend to capture the attention of the ego, or conditioned mind, activating its associational network. This can derail the deeper unconscious processing that psychedelics allow. For this reason, the therapist should avoid playing a lot of popular music. Human singing can be a potent evocator for emotion, but it's best if any song lyrics in a psychedelic playlist are in a foreign language.

Some therapists make their own playlists, either choosing songs on the fly or assembling a playlist beforehand, tailored to the client. It is best if the music is mostly new to the client, and thus less likely to evoke memories and associations that could disrupt what's happening organically. You can collaborate with the client on a playlist, selecting music that will be right for them, but it needn't all be music they like. There will surely be moments in any playlist where the client likes what they're hearing, and other times when they do not. All of this is grist for the mill, material to work with in the journey. Some clients even report that the "worst" parts of the playlist enabled the deepest work of the session. We encourage clients not to be attached to liking or not liking the music. And skipping certain tracks or stopping the playlist altogether is always an available option, if they deem it necessary.

CONCLUSION

A well-prepared journeyer is one who can safely set out on their voyage with confidence and a sense of trust. Their "backpack" has everything they need, they know the terrain, they're aware of possible pitfalls, and have contingency plans in place. Trepidation is normal—and might even be a sign of health! In fact, this fear may reassure the therapist that the client is not being cavalier about the risks and challenges of psychedelics.

The therapist should be prepared to answer all questions the client has, building trust and strengthening the container. If you're going to guide someone on a journey, it's important to screen them first, and suggest waiting if you think it could be dangerous or countertherapeutic. Make sure the client knows how difficult this work can be, and some of the risks involved. Inform them of the plan for the day, your fees and rules, your orientation to touch, and your emergency plan. Get clarity together on the choice of medicine and the dose. Ask them about their intentions and their orientation to spirituality—or lack thereof. Give them exercises for grounding and stabilization. If possible, show them the space and have them practice with any accoutrements you may be using, such as eyeshades or headphones. Most importantly, have them practice embodiment, dropping into present-tense somatic awareness.

The preparation stage is crucial in establishing a good mental *set* and creating an optimal *setting* for the journey. Focus and care during this stage can result in significantly better outcomes, avoid any number of pitfalls, and provide the journeyer with the essential sense of safety that allows these medicines to work their magic.

CHECKLIST: INTAKE

Here are some things to check for as you consider whether a prospective journeyer is ready—and, if you are a good fit to support their journey. It's always OK to tell a person "No," or to suggest they look for another practitioner:

- ☐ Why does this person want to take psychedelics at this time?
- ☐ Do they have any history with expanded states of consciousness? Has their experience been solely recreational, or have they been with a guide or therapist? How did that go?
- ☐ Have they ever had a psychotic episode? Have they been given a diagnosis of schizophrenia, bipolar I, or had incidents involving a break with reality?
- ☐ Is there any history of psychosis in their family?
- ☐ Has a mental health professional ever diagnosed them with a personality disorder? This wouldn't necessarily be a rule out but is something we should know.
- ☐ Do they have a history of trauma or chronic stress? This could be a shock trauma (a single extreme event), developmental wounding, intergenerational violence, or other kinds of overwhelming experiences that create symptoms.
- ☐ Do they tend to dissociate? How extreme are these reactions?
- ☐ How is their physical health in general? If it's been a

while, would they be willing to get a checkup from their primary care doctor before journeying with you?
- ☐ Do they have any cardiovascular issues? Journeys can be challenging for the heart, literally as well as metaphorically. Any prior issues with stroke? However healing a journey might be, the client shouldn't be risking their life for it.
- ☐ Do they have other issues with organ function? Are the liver and kidneys filtering well?
- ☐ Do they currently have suicidal ideation? Have they made suicide attempts in the past, or developed a plan and sought the means to end their life? Any disordered eating?
- ☐ Is there a somatic, mindfulness, or movement practice that they find helpful? Do they practice yoga, meditation, or breathing practices? What grounds them in times of challenge?
- ☐ Does this person have a good support system? Do they have a psychotherapist or bodyworker they see regularly? Do they have family and/or friends they trust, people they can rely on for acceptance and encouragement?

CHECKLIST: TO COMPLETE IN THE PREPARATION SESSION(S)

Though not an exhaustive list, here are some things we should be aware of as we prepare clients for psychedelic work:

- ☐ Get a signed and dated copy of your informed consent form, as well as any other forms you use in your practice.
- ☐ Take a personal history if you don't know this client. Make sure you have a plan for recordkeeping, and let the client know how you plan to handle this.

- ☐ Discuss confidentiality (including any limits to confidentiality).
- ☐ Describe your fee structure, detailing when payments are expected and what they will be.
- ☐ Get an emergency contact.
- ☐ Ask about prescriptions, supplements, or patterns of self-medicating. Explore any drug interactions that concern you (particularly SSRIs).
- ☐ Inquire into their spirituality (or lack thereof). See if there are any rituals that would feel nourishing for them. Invite them to bring personal items to create an altar (or just for comfort).
- ☐ Thoroughly discuss the possibility of touch, perhaps practicing physical contact and exploring boundaries and safety. Emphasize that this is nonsexual touch, and that consent can be withdrawn at any time.
- ☐ Teach them somatic tools for self-regulation, which could include orienting to the environment, grounding, working with the breath, and self-touch.
- ☐ If you plan to play music, discuss this with them.
- ☐ If possible, show them the room they'll be journeying in. Have them practice putting on eyeshades and headphones if they'll be used.
- ☐ Make sure you describe how challenging the work can be, and detail the risks that are unavoidably part of psychedelic exploration.
- ☐ Set ground rules. At a minimum, we suggest the following: no harm to self, no harm to the therapist, no damaging the space, and no leaving the premises until the journey is over.
- ☐ Get clear together on the medicine you'll use and dosage.
- ☐ Help them develop an intention(s) for their journey.

- ☐ Describe how important it is to trust the medicine, letting go of expectations and being open to what comes up.
- ☐ Make a comprehensive plan for the dosing session, including the approximate timing of drop-off and pickup (they won't be able to drive). Let them know what to wear, what to eat, and how to prepare on the morning of. Encourage them to leave the day(s) after the journey open, giving themselves time for physical recovery, spiritual grounding, and psychological integration.
- ☐ Schedule an integration session within the day or two following the journey.

CHAPTER 8

Designing the Space

As your environment changes, so do the neural circuits within your brain.
—IVY ROSS

When my [Manuela] client Steven first came to my office, he briefly looked around before saying, "Your space feels very nice." He exhaled, relaxed on the couch, and grabbed a fluffy pillow, holding it close to his chest for comfort. Aware of his curiosity and need for comfort, I invited him to explore the room visually. As he scanned, he spotted a Balinese statue gifted to me. His eyes rested on the figure and he smiled, commenting on how calming the statue was. As he relaxed, his eyes roamed further. He took in the details of the flower arrangement on the table, the small objects on the bookshelf, and even the wall color.

"I like that blue color," he said. "It reminds me of the ocean." After a reflective pause, he exhaled in relief. His skin became rosier, the clench of his hands eased, and he dropped further into his body. I offered, "How about making that couch yours? Do you want to stretch out or get more comfortable?" He immediately pushed off his heavy boots, stretched out on the couch, and gently closed his eyes. After a few moments, he said, "Wow, this is so different from my visit to the ketamine clinic 2 months ago. I thought I might never try this again."

Steven shared about the room where he received his first ketamine infusion, how cold and clinical it was. The sterile environment of the ketamine clinic reminded him of a hospital, he said, devoid of any inviting décor or warmth. He had expected a setting more like a therapy office, and was surprised by the medical appearance of the clinic. He struggled with the effects of ketamine and felt as if he was "sick and ill," while at the same time "tripping." The room brought back a childhood memory of being treated in a hospital, and he could not relax into the ketamine experience. He started to have a dissonant experience that elevated his anxiety.

Although kind and professional, the nurse practitioner could not ease Steven's fears. His body tensed as he waited to return to ordinary consciousness, fantasizing about leaving the clinic as quickly as possible. He concluded that ketamine was not for him and that it made him feel bad. As he stretched out on the couch, his eyes closed and he exhaled deeply, saying that if he had been in a space like this, he would not have felt so disconnected.

Where and how we journey has a profound impact on the experience itself. We have described set and setting as crucial determinants of therapeutic journeys. While *setting* can be defined as the physical space the journey takes place in, it could also include the social and cultural environment (Hartogsohn, 2017). Clients pick up on religious or social undertones, beliefs, and attitudes around drugs in general, as well as whether the space supports a more psychotherapeutic experience or an experiential one (Hartogsohn, 2020). In general, the setting should be a healing space removed from familiar distractions and intrusions—one that allows the client's journey to become sacred and intentional. The setting plays a role in whether the psychedelic experience is a powerful and safe expansion or a fearful, negative contraction (Leary et al., 1992).

This chapter explores how therapists can create a practical, comfortable, inviting, and effective therapy space. Sacred space needs tending: Your presence, attention to detail, and care will make all the difference in the atmosphere. This is not about buying expensive furniture or art, but the mindful placement of meaningful objects. It is about creating flow in the office that allows the body to move and be comfortable, supporting the client's physical, social, and psychological needs (Aixalà, 2022).

Setting isn't just a clinical consideration. Indigenous cultures have understood the importance of physical space as an elemental aspect of psychedelic work. Traditionally, ayahuasca ceremonies are held in the jungle, in resonance with nature. In Indigenous and First Nations communities, sacred ceremonies are deeply interwoven with ritual, community, and the natural world. In Mazatec ceremonies, the night ritual, *velada*, is conducted with divination practices, chants, prayers, and purifications with copal smoke to set the scene for the impending journey (Fagetti & Mercadillo, 2022). The setting itself is a gateway to the expansion of consciousness. In Indigenous ceremonial practices, the physical space and setting are integral to the safety, spiritual connection, cultural context, and overall efficacy of the psychedelic experience. The setting—often handed down through the generations—is carefully chosen to honor tradition and lineage, facilitate spiritual growth and energetic protection, and promote harmony with nature. Rivers, forests, and mountains hold cultural and spiritual significance for these ceremonies and support spiritual leaders in their work.

THE NEUROAESTHETIC SPACE

Artists and healers have long understood that ritual, dance, and song need to be held in sacred spaces, environments that nurture the human quest to touch the divine within. Beauty and aesthetics enhance our relationship with the immediate environment. Visual art, music, and dance have a multidimensional impact on our psychological, spiritual, and physiological health. Visual processing is central to the human experience. In fact, more than 50% of the brain's outer surface, the cortex, is dedicated to vision (Van Essen, 2003), and the brain has two distinct networks for processing visual inputs (Milner & Goodale, 2008).

We vigilantly scan for safety and are soothed by a colorful painting or nature-scape. Our parasympathetic "rest and digest" system calms us when we perceive beauty and harmony in the natural world: a spiral pattern in tree bark, a bright flower, or the saturated blue of the ocean.

Thanks to the field of *neuroaesthetics*, which studies the biological underpinnings of the pleasure and meaning we derive from aesthetic objects and experiences, we know humans have an innate desire for beauty. Susan Magsamen (2019), founder of the Arts and Mind Lab at John Hopkins University School of Medicine, argues that our thirst for aesthetic experiences is hardwired. How healing spaces are designed—and whether they follow trauma-informed principles—can impact patients' nervous systems.

Neuroaesthetic considerations, such as how we perceive safety, beauty, and pleasure, have been implemented in many healing spaces to decrease anxiety and agitation. For example, many pediatric hospitals or oncology wings have quiet, inviting spaces with natural lighting, comfortable seating, and greenery. Intentionally designed homeless shelters and affordable housing zones include green spaces, as well as architectural features with curves—as primates, we prefer natural shapes and smooth arcs that mimic plants and animals rather than hard, sharp edges (Kourtzi & Connor, 2011). Studies have shown that when art therapies are part of treatment they reduce stress (Kaimal et al., 2016), improve cognitive abilities (Shukla et al., 2022), and show great promise in treating trauma (Schouten et al., 2014).

CONNECTION TO NATURE

Studies in public health, urban planning, sustainability, and ecotherapy have concluded that exposure to nature can reduce trauma symptoms and decrease stress (Berman et al., 2008; Bratman et al., 2012). One study found that when residents of disadvantaged areas were exposed to green spaces, their stress response was significantly reduced (Hunter et al., 2019). Watering of plants and light gardening help reduce blood pressure and change brain-wave activity, calming us (Hassan & Deshun, 2023).

A study of military veterans with PTSD found that engaging in outdoor activities—such as angling, equine care, and archery—significantly reduced PTSD symptoms and improved overall psychological health (Wheeler et al., 2020). Conducted as a pilot study and a randomized controlled trial, the research demonstrated that these activities not only decreased PTSD symptoms but also enhanced social functioning and reduced depression, anxiety, and perceived stress, showcasing the therapeutic potential of nature-based interventions for veterans with PTSD.

Further research indicates that bringing elements of nature indoors can provide significant mental health benefits, particularly for individuals who have experienced trauma. For example, exposure to natural environments can reduce symptoms of anxiety, depression, and PTSD, and these benefits can be replicated to some extent with indoor nature exposure. For example, Gregory Bratman and colleagues (2021) highlight that exposure to nature, both outdoors and indoors—such as through plants, natural light, and images of natural scenes—can help reduce stress, improve mood, and enhance cognitive function. Their work demonstrates that activities like walking in natural environments can decrease negative thinking patterns (rumination) and increase positive affect.

I [Manuela] saw the importance of a natural connection firsthand. My client, Lena, walked into my small San Francisco office and was immediately grief-stricken at the sight before her. "How could you move that plant without my consent?" she blurted out. This was in my first city office, where I began my clinical practice. A beautiful ficus plant had grown so large it covered the natural light and cut the small, expensive urban space in half. Unbeknownst to me, Lena had bonded with the thriving tree. That day, I realized the office wasn't just mine. It belonged to my clients' dreams, experiences, and expectations—it was a community space. Lena grieved the loss of this plant every time she came for her sessions. Weeks later, I returned the tree, wedging it into its familiar tight place.

Psychedelic journeys can help clients reflect on their relationship with nature (Kettner et al., 2019). As part of the well-known effect of *ego dissolution*, psychedelic journeyers may relax and experience an energetic feeling of being held, of belonging. A central theme for many clients is mourning their lack of emotional connection with nature, the loss of feeling the biosphere as a direct ally. Other times, a sense of kinship with the natural world can become a profound resource. One of my clients described a highlight moment in their journey as "being part of nature," as if nature was not something distinctly different from their body.

Bringing elements of the natural world into the physical therapy setting—literally or symbolically—is advised. This can help create a warm holding space. It can reduce anxiety, bringing mental and physical equilibrium to the client. In the psychedelic journey, an essential aspect is to feel safe and held so that challenging experiences can be experienced with less resistance, and natural elements in the setting can help.

THE BODY NEEDS TO MOVE

In somatic therapy work, it can be supportive to encourage clients to move their bodies and vocalize. This contrasts with some models of psychedelic-assisted therapy, in which the client is instructed to lie on a bed, remaining still and focusing on thoughts and feelings. In some ceremonial rituals, also, participants are encouraged to stay on their mats and contain their physical expression. There may be valid and important considerations for this. Yet, in somatic psychedelic work, we want movement to be possible. The client might need more room for their body to move.

This ability, to move the body—stretching, swaying, pushing, rolling, and rhythmically expressing our attunement to music or internal cues—can allow for important somatic openings and transformative experiences. New neurological patterns can be wired in when a journeyer performs catlike stretches that open the chest. Strong emotions can be released and metabolized by allowing the arms and legs to move. For some, societal oppression has resulted in physical constriction: The body is small, stiff, and bound. These clients might feel further contraction when asked to lie still. If the physical space does not have enough room to move, it can send an unconscious message to the client that body movement and freedom are not allowed.

Physical space, and how we set it up, communicates ideas and expectations about how bodies are allowed to be. Most clients don't make large movements—but sometimes the body yearns to stretch, undulate, dance, crawl, or roll on the ground. If the space is there, the body will know how to inhabit it. If the space is not inviting for the body, self-expression may be inhibited. We should want to invite the whole human experience, allowing the expansion not just of the mind but also the body.

DESIGNING A TRAUMA-INFORMED AND NEUROAESTHETIC SPACE

We often think of designing space as putting in "stuff"—a couch, a color scheme, objects—without considering the objects' energy, history, or provenance. Are the pieces there simply because they look good, or are they connected to places? Do they have meaning, or come with a rich story? What does the object represent? A clinical, tame space devoid of color—or one that contains objects intended to be neutral—can be as alienating to the client as a randomly furnished space designed without much consideration.

The brain becomes sensitive to interoceptive and exteroceptive influences in the expanded state. If we don't feel safe in the journey, the body will respond with tension—and, possibly, be triggered into a stress response. How our body perceives the immediate surroundings is highly subjective and based on prior experience. This is often unconscious. We don't typically think that the physical environment can substantially influence our inner state, though the field of *environmental psychology* has demonstrated over and over that it does.

I [Manuela] attended a session in a ketamine clinic and noticed that the clinicians had placed affirmations around the room. "You can do it," "Just breathe," "Home is where you belong," "You are home," and other peppy messages were artfully scattered across the walls. The messages on neon plastic signs were intended to be positive and uplifting, yet I wondered about the subliminal messages being delivered. I felt I was being told how I should feel, and my body's initial response was to recoil. *What if I don't feel at home? What does that even mean?* I was immediately forced to confront a theme generated from the outside rather than from within. Did I need that much encouragement for my imminent ketamine session? The neon signs swirled in my head as I embarked on my journey.

There are currently two main approaches when designing the psychedelic office space. One is to make the room as neutral as possible, with no "offensive" art, religious symbols, or bright colors. The idea is that the client has a blank canvas on which to project their own psychic experience. The other approach is personalizing the therapy room, reflecting the therapist's unique character. I have heard psychedelic therapist colleagues refer to the office as their personal space, reflecting their unique lineage and intention. Regardless of whether the space is neutral or uniquely personalized, the therapist should be aware of the setting's impact on the client's need for safety, comfort, and a feeling of welcome. Anything placed within view of the client should be carefully considered from the perspective of the psychedelic journeyer. Even seemingly innocuous objects can have an unintended impact.

CREATE AN AWAKE SACRED SPACE

Bringing sacredness to your environment is about bringing heart and presence to it. In the secular *Shambhala* approach, influenced by Tibetan Buddhism, this teaching is called *drala* (Trungpa, 1984). *Drala* is the sacred energy that is always present in our world, awake and open, and we can access that reverent energy if given the right supports. In our physical space, a dry plant neglected in the corner is *negative drala*. In contrast, a simple, carefully placed, freshly cut flower can evoke an "awake" quality in the space, which is *positive drala*.

Creating an awake sacred space is about presence. We consider how the space will appear to the client. The incorporation of objects evoking positive *drala*, such as a candle, flowers, or objects with personal meaning, will facilitate an easy entry into expanded states of consciousness—in ways that a collection of decorative religious or spiritual symbols can never do. In other words, *awake sacred space* is not about the stuff you accumulate but how you place and relate to objects as an expression of awake presence.

Awake sacred spaces invite the journeyer to cross into hallowed ground through the portals of perception. It should be a quiet space that calls for introspection and contemplation; when the client walks in, it should feel as if they are transitioning into a different space. The body recognizes sacredness in many environments, such as a church, a temple, a group of trees, a canyon, a hut in the jungle, a forest, or a carefully tended office space.

Antelope Canyon is one such majestic, awake sacred space. It is a wind- and water-swept slot canyon in the Arizona desert that has long been a sacred site of the Navajo Nation. To experience its magic, the visitor descends a ladder into a steep canyon and navigates narrow, curved passageways of sensuous red, yellow, and pink sandstone, shimmering in the sunlight. Called Tsé Bíghanílíní by the Navajo, which means "the place where water runs through rocks," the dramatic curves and intricate patterns of the sandstone were created by water and compressed over millions of years into undulating walls. The Navajo believe that spiritual beings called *hózhó*, representing beautiful harmony and balance, dwell at this sacred site. When walking in the slot canyon, the breeze moves quietly through the winding landscape, and the sun's brilliance illuminates the bright red and orange color and smooth texture of the rocks. Witnessing the sheer beauty of nature's magnificence, one finds awe here. This awake sacred space opens a remembrance: sacred *drala* invites the traveler to remember where they belong. We can bring the inspiration we feel in such places into our indoor environments, allowing ourselves to be guided as we arrange and decorate the space.

Invite Somatic Movement

To create a setting that allows your client to express themselves through their body, you can consider having a mattress on the floor rather than on a raised frame. This allows the journeyer to roll onto the floor and move easily if needed. A carpeted space feels welcoming. Pillows, blankets, soft surfaces, and pleasing textures invite the client to move and participate in the journey.

If you do somatic movement work, you want the space to accommodate easy transitions from lying down to stretching or rolling on the carpet. If you set up a bed, ensure you have room to sit next to the client at a comfortable distance, allowing you to get around and tend to their needs. Create a space that is accessible for all body types and abilities. Some clients can't lie down on the ground, and planning for these needs is part of the design. Create a clean space where you can sit next to the client on the floor (ideally, on a floor chair, such as a "BackJack"); if you have a bed, make sure you have a comfortable chair for yourself. If you have a hybrid space with a designated somatic movement space, make sure you have that set up beforehand. Explain that space to the client and how they will transition there when necessary. This might involve physically helping them, so make this as easy as possible. When you move from the couch or bed to the floor, set this up to ensure you have everything you need (such as blankets, pillows, tissues, etc.). When you change your physical location in the session, be mindful that physical positions might shift; you might be closer to the client and will need to be conscious of reestablishing energetic boundaries. You might have several sitting areas in a somatic movement space to accommodate the client's movement around the room. For example, you might have a meditation cushion, a floor chair next to a mattress on the floor, and an armchair (or two, if you are working with a co-therapist) next to a sofa or bed.

Invite Nature

Create an environment that symbolizes a connection with nature. Freshly cut flowers and potted plants uplift the environment. Nature images on the wall or nature sculptures can also be a reminder of the natural world. A water feature—such as a small fountain, or images of a river or the sea—can also stimulate that connection. You can invite clients to bring an element from nature to place on an altar. As much as possible, use natural, diffuse, soft lighting. If you have access to green space from your office, that is a bonus. Your clients will enjoy a view of a tree, a glimpse of the sky, or access to a garden after their journey.

Consider Colors and Textures

As you design the space, consider the color palette. It should incorporate inviting and pleasing tones. Choose warm colors and ambient lighting, if possible. Add texture and interest to your space, reflecting your environment and uniqueness. It should be engaging enough for others to feel comfortable.

Create an aesthetically pleasing space with artwork that is meaningful and inspiring. Place objects, perhaps meaningful ones, that can serve as gentle reminders for the journey. Be careful with religious symbols as they can be alienating to clients. You want the space to exude a mixture of warmth and comfort so the client does not feel overwhelmed by the therapist's personality. Be mindful of objects you bring in that have personal meaning for you and examine what will be inviting for a client. I once subleased an office space from a colleague in which all their shamanic travel artifacts were on display. The first impression was that of a museum, with colorful masks and psychedelic cultural artifacts mixed with religious symbols collected worldwide. My clients felt intimidated and distracted by the cluttered space. If in doubt, have a friend sit in your space and ask them if they feel they could make this space their own—or whether they feel like a guest in someone's house.

Ensure Physical Comfort and Safety

Set up your space with physical safety in mind, ensuring there are no sharp corners, fragile objects, or items that could be tripped on. Make the room clutter-free so you and the client won't have to worry about bumping into anything. Ensure there is easy access to a private bathroom. Consider privacy in the space, such as a window covering, to make sure your client will not feel exposed in front of a window or a door opening.

Have ample clean and comfortable pillows and blankets. Their temperature might change dramatically, so having blankets of varying thicknesses would be helpful. Have a weighted blanket for clients who want to be held and cocooned. Place a heater or fan nearby to cater to the client's temperature needs.

Remind your client to wear (or bring) comfortable, breathable, natural fibers and clothes they can move in freely. Layers are good. Avoid buttons and zippers. Bring a change of clothing for after the journey, as the body might go through temperature changes.

Limit Outside Noise but Add Music

Your space should be quiet and relatively free of noise and distractions. If the room is not soundproof, consider adding a sound machine or investing in soundproofing for the walls so extraneous sounds won't be heard and vocalizations or music won't travel outside. Music is the *hidden therapist* (Kaelen et al., 2018) for the psychedelic journey and can be very important. Prepare your space with a sound system and music playlists you are familiar with. Have your music ready and tailored to your client's needs. Invest time in creating lists of music, as understanding the arc of a session and the flow of music that will support the journey is an art.

CREATING RITUAL SPACE

An altar is a simple reflection of a sacred space; having one in the therapy setting can be a thoughtful touch. It is a reminder that you are tending to the *drala* of the space, bringing in an awake focus. You can designate a small table or a shelf for this purpose. A candle, a flower, photos, divination cards, a ritual object that holds spiritual import for you, or a meaningful object that matches the client's intentions can be placed on the altar. Invite the client to bring anything that symbolizes a sacred space for them.

We often create altars with my client's journey in mind. The altar might include a beautiful cloth, a fresh candle that we can gift to the client after, a simple flower, or a small nature arrangement to create a focal point. We then add objects depending on what has been prepared with the client. For example, if they are working on the theme of embodiment and safety, they could hold a rock or connect with soothing herbs burning or steeping in the room; if the client is seeking spiritual connection, we might ask them to bring a figurine or image that symbolizes their spiritual beliefs. As you cocreate the altar, encourage mindful reflection on what has meaning for them and what connects with their intentions for the session.

For your own spiritual connection or grounding, you can have objects that have meaning for you on the altar—and consider bringing rituals and prayers into the overall experience. Use discretion when sharing these personal items and rituals. These mindful intentions invoke sacred space, marking the transition from ordinary interaction to inner exploration. Include an awareness of cultural sensitivity and inclusivity—you want to anticipate what may be inviting or alienating to your client. Use your intuition and the knowledge of the client from the preparation session(s) to determine this. Journeyers can feel uncomfortable with rituals and objects that have no meaning to them, and might feel less grounded as a result.

Have the client sit quietly before ingesting the medicine to reflect on their intentions. A few moments of mindful awareness, spent connecting to intentions and centering bodily presence, are essential optimizers for the mystical experience. Singing, drumming, or moving mindfully were traditionally used to prepare the setting, creating a connection with sacred aspects within (Winkelman, 2021). If you're not already part of one of these traditions, you can still incorporate this wisdom.

Try This: Owning the Space and Intention Setting

1. Invite your client to practice looking around the room briefly. This orienting practice will help settle their nervous system and allow them to "own the space."
2. As the client orients in the room, track their body and notice whether their breathing rhythm settles and calms.
3. Guide them as they slowly look around the room. You can say, "Go ahead and see what you like in this room. What speaks to you right now? What do you need to get fully

comfortable here? What is it like for you to take this time and fully arrive? Is there anything you want to change?"
4. Then, ask the client to set a simple and positive intention for their journey. Remind them to keep it short and focus on a purpose rather than a goal.
5. Ask them to let go and enter the journey with an open attitude, readying themselves to receive what emerges.

CLEANSING THE SPACE

A clean space is both physically and energetically clean. I remember having a session with a psychedelic guide who had fully booked her week with back-to-back clients. When I entered the space, she hastily turned over the sheets on the mat, picking up tissues and water glasses from the session before. The space was visually beautiful but needed to be cared for and made ready for me. It had not been energetically cleansed from the previous sessions, and a heaviness hung in the air. I could feel a contraction in my body and I did not feel welcomed.

Indigenous shamans, as part of creating sacred space, will bless and purify the ceremony that is about to take place. Before entering the space, careful rituals are performed to cleanse it with sacred plants, such as palo santo and sage, calling forth protective spirits and purifying any negative energies. The shaman often calls on spiritual allies and elemental forces to aid their work, praying for their help to protect the ceremony from outside interference (Gonzalez et al., 2021).

In many indigenous traditions, secret rituals, ceremonial herbs, music, and prayers are also used to cleanse the person entering. Being on a preparatory diet, setting intentions, paying attention to the body and mental processes—all of these are part of honoring sacred space. The participant may be cleansed with smoke, prayers, and plants, connecting them to the ceremonial setting. A connection to nature—to the rivers, mountains, and forests—is also called upon.

CONCLUSION

Effectively designing a space is essential, nonverbally communicating to journeyers that they are held in safety. Creating an intentional environment will facilitate the client's transition into a productive therapeutic space, one that integrates elements of the sacred and makes it meaningful for the journeyer. Design a comfortable and practical setting to meet the client's physical and emotional needs. Feeling held is paramount in the journey. This begins with the setting, which creates an optimal mental set and allows deep work to emerge. Make your physical space inviting so that you—and your client—feel at home.

CHECKLIST: SOMATIC PSYCHEDELIC-FRIENDLY OFFICE SPACE AND SUPPLIES

Here is a checklist of what would help set up your somatic-friendly space and the supplies you should have ready for your work:

- ☐ Designate an open, uncluttered space, without any obstructions (such as chairs or furniture). This area can be an open carpet spot, or a place where you have removed furniture.
- ☐ Have a comfortable, clean carpet, a mat, or a thick blanket ready so you can invite the client to do floor work. Also, have a floor chair nearby so you can easily shift support positions.

- ☐ Have extra pillows with different types of support. Soft pillows that invite touch, which clients can hold and cuddle, can be helpful (especially for people who are averse to physical touch). Sturdy pillows should be on hand in case the client wants to hit or kick.
- ☐ Have a variety of blankets available. The client's body temperature will fluctuate, so having both light and heavyweight, cozy blankets is helpful. Have weighted blankets available for clients who need containment and soothing and don't want to be touched.
- ☐ Depending on the client's temperature needs, a fan and/or heater can modulate the temperature to keep them cool or warm.
- ☐ Have dimmable lights and create unobtrusive lighting (lamps and natural sources of light are generally preferred over overhead fixtures).
- ☐ Consider privacy. For example, ensure that your client will not feel exposed in front of a window or door. Soundproof if necessary.
- ☐ Consider your client's physical abilities and make accommodations in advance. Be prepared so you will not have to make last-minute adjustments to the space.
- ☐ Ensure that a private bathroom is accessible for your client. Create ambient lighting in the bathroom, and make sure they have tissues and clean facial towels available to use.
- ☐ Eyeshades. Many clients have a preferred eyeshade, which you can ask them to bring. Have some of your own handy, and ensure they are clean and made from natural fibers (cotton or silk).
- ☐ Art or drawing supplies. The client might like to draw or write in preparation or after, so have some art materials, a writing pad, and pens nearby.

- ☐ Try to have a physio ball (exercise or yoga ball), stretch bands, and foam rollers to move or stretch. This can be helpful for embodiment during the preparation phase, or used when the client is waiting for the medicine to take effect. Some clients appreciate gentle stretching and movement to metabolize anxiety and deepen their connection with the body. These props are also helpful after a session and during integration.
- ☐ Headphones for music. Over-ear headphones are more comfortable and reliable for clients during the journey. A sound system that can be heard simultaneously in the room and in headphones is ideal. You can research the best systems and setups that would work for your office.
- ☐ Have your music playlist prepared (and be ready to change the music if necessary). Having the right music takes preparation and care. Spend some time researching music for your practice.
- ☐ Some additional items that might be useful: soft facial tissues, a spillproof water bottle, and a bowl or wastebasket for purging (with a washcloth or small towel nearby).

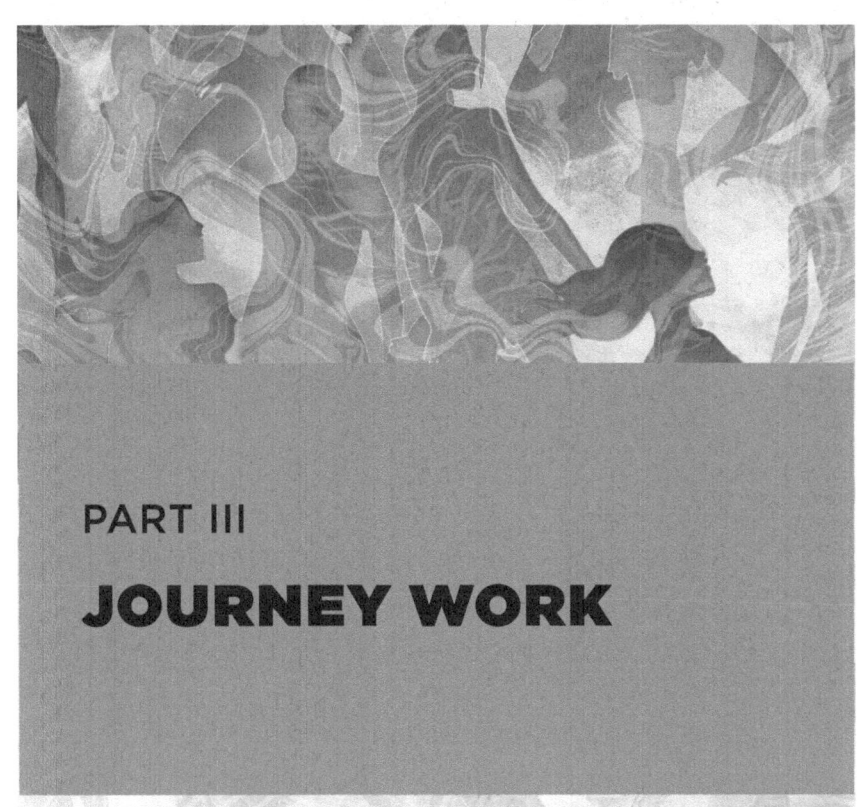

PART III

JOURNEY WORK

CHAPTER 9
Embodied Journeys

From wonder into wonder existence opens.
—LAO TZU

Psychedelic intoxication is a realm unto itself. In conventional therapy, we steadily work against habits of body and mind to make change possible. This can take a long time, requiring weeks, months, or years of diligent work. But in psychedelic journeys, new pathways arise spontaneously in vivid explosions of color, visceral sensations, and novel insights. Whereas massage therapists coax muscle and fascia into alignment, and psychotherapists challenge the mind to discover fresh perspectives, the psychedelic therapist need only administer a dose and await a flurry of new experiences. Again, this is not healing in and of itself. The psychedelic experience must be examined and integrated afterward. However, practitioners accustomed to slow and steady progress toward therapeutic goals—with regular setbacks—may be stunned to see the way altered states of consciousness can beget sudden and immediate shifts.

The principle of *emergence* comes into play here. Emergence describes the way complex systems suddenly reveal unpredictable properties, sometimes called the *butterfly effect* (Lorenz, 1972). The simple building blocks of a system can come together in unforeseen ways, which give rise to unpredictable phenomena. The behavior of an individual ant, for instance, does nothing to suggest the labyrinthine structure of an anthill, with thousands of workers cooperating in sophisticated ways. Similarly, the psyche may weave its healing from a variegated tapestry of experience, which appears inscrutable to the observer. The client may not be expecting anything like this, but the therapist's readiness for the unexpected can send a calming signal. It is the clinician's responsibility to avoid directing the process.

THE PHASES OF A PSYCHEDELIC JOURNEY

The first stage of any psychedelic experience is ingestion. Often, therapists develop rituals for this, presenting the material to the client in a special bowl, glass, or pot. A ceremonial aspect to this first encounter with the medicine is not uncommon, perhaps involving the utterance of a particular phrase—or an invitation to observe a moment of silence—before it is taken.

The psychedelic experience then progresses in a kind of arc: a predictable series of phases. Familiarity with this structure can help therapists plan the course of the day, select music appropriate to each phase, and anticipate how things may unfold. Bonny and Pahnke (1972) first described this sequence, though the specific terms we use come from Kaelen et al. (2018):

> *Pre-onset* is the time after the administration of a psychedelic, but before any drug effects are perceptible. The therapist's job during this phase is to simply help the journeyer relax, establishing a mental set conducive to a therapeutic journey.
> *Onset* is when the journeyer first begins to feel high. For some, this transition may cause anxiety, especially if the

client is unaccustomed to altered states. In this phase, the therapist can provide reassurance that things are progressing on course, normalizing the journeyer's experience, and using somatic tracking to help them "go with the flow."

Building toward peak is when drug effects steadily climb in intensity, demanding a deeper letting go on the part of the journeyer. Visual hallucinations and somatosensory distortions often begin at this phase, with cognition and spatial orientation growing more and more strange. The therapist may become less involved here, as the rush of inner phenomena begins to capture the journeyer's attention.

Peak is the point when drug effects are strongest. Here the journeyer is fully subsumed in the psychedelic experience, which may bring feelings of acute vulnerability, emotional release, ego dissolution, or other transcendent states of illumination. This is a good time to cue the most powerful and evocative music in the playlist. The client may reach out for more connection as they navigate the intensity of the peak, yet they may also lose facility with language or motor function, and become incapable of asking directly for our help. The therapist can offer a supportive touch to steady the client as they surf the biggest waves of their journey.

Reentry is more commonly known as the comedown. As drug effects diminish, the observing ego comes back online and journeyers begin to feel like themselves again. There is often a sense of snapping back to "normal," and they may become chatty and distracted. However, the journey is by no means over yet. Therapists can encourage clients to make the most of this liminal time, staying inwardly focused and present with the flow of experience, as important work can still occur in this phase.

Return is the final phase, where the journeyer lands back in an ordinary state of consciousness. Some clients may be relieved the experience has ended, while others may be despondent. The therapist's objective is to welcome the person back, celebrating their courage and resilience through the day's ordeal and helping them adjust to feeling normal again. We should dissuade them from analyzing the journey right away, and instead encourage reorientation and settling. A light snack, such as sliced fruit or warm broth, may help ground the client, as well as provide them with some much-needed calories. It's important to note that tinges of psychedelic effects may still be present, including sensory distortions—journeyers should refrain from operating a vehicle, responding to emails, or attending to any other routine obligations.

The length of these phases varies depending on the specific type of medicine. Additionally, people have different constitutions and process drugs at different rates. Some may enter the *onset* phase more quickly than others, or reach the *peak* sooner and stay there longer. We can't know exactly how things will play out. Having a rough approximation of the journey's arc, though, will prepare us for what's to come.

NONLINEARITY

Predictable phases notwithstanding, one should anticipate nonlinearity in psychedelic experiences. Intensity may ebb and flow, and people may unpredictably feel more or less altered for seemingly no reason. The time course may be different for every person, as will the content.

As the anarchic brain takes hold, journeyers may hop around from theme to theme in a seemingly chaotic way. This erraticism may have an intelligence concealed within it, though, and the therapist should not try to impose order.

Journeyers often explore the timeline of their lives in a nonlinear fashion. They might at one moment remember a recent conversation, which links a dimly remembered feeling from childhood, which then leads to the recall of an event from adolescence. The psyche combs through the accumulated history of a lifetime, seeking out moments of unprocessed experience. The client may express emotions that were repressed, allow the body to complete motor actions or postures that were previously inhibited, or receive latent insights that were awaiting discovery.

Eastern wisdom traditions might describe this process as purifying one's *karma*. Westerners often simplistically interpret karma as "what goes around, comes around," a cosmic scorecard in which one is punished for misdeeds and rewarded for selfless action. However, a truer description of karma might be one's *unlived life*.

We carry around experiences we have not fully felt and integrated, which may affect the course of our lives. For example, if I harm another person, but never allow myself to move through an empathic response of guilt, my prospects in life could be diminished. I will unconsciously manifest this burden of shame in my dealings with others. The resulting distortion in my self-concept creates a tendency to draw negative outcomes toward myself. These imprints are often assimilated in psychedelic sessions, as the journeyer completes whatever past experiences they had not previously made room for.

Because the journey is nonlinear, therapists must continually coach their clients, as well as themselves, to avoid judging what happens. The part of the brain that judges and tries to control experience—in both the therapist and the journeyer—should be quieted during the dosing session. We can't predict what will happen, and may be humbled to see the principle of emergence in action. The flap of a butterfly's wings in Brazil could indeed set off a tornado in Texas. A seemingly random image or sensation—or disconnected thought, or feeling—arising in a chaotic way may lead to a profound understanding for the journeyer. The therapist must go with the flow of the session, not imposing interpretations too quickly, or approaching the journey like a puzzle to be solved.

This nondirective approach can feel counterintuitive to mental health professionals, or to people who like to problem solve and make sense of things. Frankly, the work can be boring for some practitioners, especially those accustomed to conducting manualized therapy sessions or applying a prescriptive protocol. But the therapist's capacity to witness and receive the journeyer without judgment is what fosters healing. We must cultivate an attitude of receptivity, a willingness to encounter whatever arises in the client's body and mind.

MINDFULNESS

Mindfulness practices will prove helpful in psychedelic therapy. Doing little more than attentive sitting for hours, the therapist may become physically antsy or mentally ruminative. The ability to still one's mind and body is important for this work. Many therapists, guides, and sitters find practices that involve tracking the breath, sensing the body, and attending to the external environment serve them well. Cultivating mindful attention to the present moment, therapists can notice what interferes with their receptivity. Distractedness *will* happen, but with greater awareness it can be recognized more quickly. The therapist can then ground and come back to center, opening their awareness, holding a sense of curiosity about what comes next for the journeyer.

Another crucial skill for psychedelic therapy is attunement. The therapist supports the journeyer by matching them. Clients respond positively to people they're simpatico with, who *get* them, and who relate in a way that is authentic. Therapists will find they have a hard time manufacturing this. Even if they try, people on psychedelics generally have a good "bullshit detector," and will know immediately if the therapist is playacting. A better approach is to simply let oneself be moved by the client's process. This often results in spontaneous entrainment, with the therapist's psycho-biological experience impacting the client in what is sometimes called a *relational field* (mentioned in Chapter 6).

THE JOINING PRINCIPLE

A key to conceptualizing therapeutic attunement is the *joining principle*. When the therapist successfully joins the journeyer, they establish a sense of shared experience, an alliance built on rapport. To do this they must avoid the extremes of merging, on the one hand, and distancing, on the other.

If the therapist starts to lose themselves in the client's process, they won't be able to contain what's happening in the session. If things feel too personal, or if we get overly involved in the client's material, it helps to focus our attention inwardly for a while. Taking time to stabilize ourselves in these moments can make all the difference, remembering that we have a body and that we're separate and distinct from the person we're supporting.

Conversely, at times the therapist might pull away. Perhaps the material emerging from the journeyer triggers us, resulting in judgment or a feeling of inadequacy. If we get overly centered on ourselves, it similarly hinders the therapeutic potential of the session. Attending outwardly can help in such moments. Coming back into awareness of the person we're supporting, sending compassionate attention their way, is important to reinstate attunement and relationship.

Are you a person who tends to merge with others, or do you tend to be more distanced? When talking with a friend—or conducting a therapy session—do you find it difficult to be present because you're having strong empathic reactions? Perhaps you want to hurt the person who bothered your friend or client, or you may feel crushed by what's saddened them.

Or, on the other hand, do you lose track of what people are saying because there's a *lack* of emotional resonance? Do you analyze them and judge their reaction to something, convinced you need to come up with a fix for their issue?

We all have our tendencies to either merge or distance. Hopefully, rather than shaming ourselves for these tendencies—compensatory patterns likely developed in early childhood—we might instead bring awareness to these habits of mind, allowing us to more easily see when they're impeding our ability to be present.

COUNTERTRANSFERENCE

The therapist may experience strong emotional reactions to a client in response to specific cues, even if this isn't their usual response. Perhaps the client mentions an issue that personally torments the therapist, or describes an event the therapist has also lived through. Journeyers may remind the therapist of figures from their past, perhaps people who wounded them (or who they idealized). Ultimately, we may not know why a client evokes such strong feelings—or creates a sense of boredom or antipathy. In the psychoanalytic tradition, these responses are called *countertransference*.

Countertransference is the converse of transference, described in Chapter 7. Whereas in transference a *client* transfers feelings and dynamics from past relationships onto the current relationship with the therapist, countertransference describes the way the *therapist* is affected by a client. Human beings evoke unconscious reactions in us, and part of the therapist's task is to see how we respond, inquiring into this internal attitude and anticipating how it could affect the work.

As we make this inquiry, it may be useful to differentiate between *objective countertransference*—feelings about a client that we could reasonably expect most people to have—and *subjective countertransference*—a personal reaction that is unique to us (Geltner, 2012). For instance, some clients are combative and rude, defending themselves against vulnerability at any cost. This can cause therapists to feel stifled, frustrated, and impatient. Most therapists would probably feel some version of these things when interacting with that particular client. On the other hand, the person seeking my help might leave me feeling irritated, or intensely guarded, for no discernible reason. They may look like a figure from my past, or have an affectation or manner of speech that reminds me of someone I detest. I could feel uncomfortable in their presence without knowing why, until I explore the subtleties of what they bring up for me. Most other therapists wouldn't have this response. I can recognize that it's my personal history restricting my ability to truly see the client. We must work through our subjective countertransference to better support those we serve.

Of course, countertransference can also be positive. Perhaps the client reminds me of a younger version of myself, or elicits attraction (this *erotic countertransference* is the inverse of the erotic transference described in Chapter 2). Positive countertransference can interfere in beneficial outcomes too. For example, the therapist may feel an unusually strong protectiveness, shielding the client from painful truths about themselves; or, they may idealize them, missing the shadow elements trying to find the light of consciousness. Cultivating awareness of all these various countertransference reactions can open the way for self-understanding in the therapist, creating greater receptivity and attunement—and more effective clinical practice.

Ultimately, much of the healing power of the therapeutic relationship comes from the therapist's ability to access compassion. It could be that the client discovers their inner healing intelligence only when they are adequately supported by another. Once someone shows up to support them, see them, and receive them, their psyche can access untapped inner strength and find new paths to transformation. A cornerstone of *humanistic*, or *person-centered psychology*, is what Carl Rogers (2012) called *unconditional positive regard*. As the practitioner rests into this stance of expansive beneficence—an acceptance and celebration of this unique person before us—the client's latent healing capacities are activated.

PSYCHEDELICS AND THE UNCONSCIOUS

Psychedelics give us direct access to the unconscious. Psychology has long recognized that conscious awareness is but a pale sliver of our total mental activity. Our thinking, feeling, and behavior are driven, conditioned, and constrained, limited by our genetic inheritance and what we learned earlier in life. On psychedelics, unconscious habits of mind are laid bare. Clients may suddenly see the assumptions and expectations that restrict them. They are now able to analyze these tendencies and see how they create their life circumstances. A person may recoil in horror at a new awareness of selfishness or sadism, or discover a wellspring of latent love and goodwill.

In this encounter, we may find the hidden parts of ourselves that we don't like and have disowned (what Jung [1951/1968] called the *shadow*), or discover what Chögyam Trungpa Rinpoche (1984) called *basic goodness*. Either way, journeyers are often surprised and delighted at the sudden rush of insight that psychedelics release. They can now see the programs running—or attempting to run—under the surface, and report a deeper connection to themselves, underneath these programs, a sense of congruence with who they truly are at their very core.

Unconscious processing relates directly to the body. Psychedelics can immerse us in a state of deep physical relaxation. As the medicine exerts its effect, journeyers may experience their bodies melting, or trembling as the body releases stored tension. This allows them to experience new ways of inhabiting the body, and in turn, new ways of being. They may find themselves suddenly seeing with new eyes, considering things from novel perspectives, feeling compassion for others (even those they've felt harmed by), and processing through emotions and thoughts about past experiences. This profound transformation of awareness results from being with the body in a different way.

This transformation facilitates disidentification from the ego, the illusory experience of being a fixed, separate self. One's personality is not just neural firing but is a somatically integrated process reflected in posture and tension patterns. The state of our body radiates up and out, determining our psychological state in a bottom-up way. Or, as Gestalt theorists Perls et al. (1951) wrote, "The neurotic personality *creates* its symptoms by *unaware manipulation of muscles*" (p. 87). The psychedelic therapist can support the soma to relax and open through touch, gentle massage, or invitations to notice the body and find more comfortable positions to sit or lie down in.

Freud (1899/1913) famously called dreams "the *via regia* to a knowledge of the unconscious" (p. 483; *via regia* is usually translated as "royal road"). If dreams are the royal road, psychedelics may be the *superhighway* to the unconscious. Journeyers often marvel at the naked transparency of their mind on psychedelics. In an inward-focused therapeutic journey, a client may suddenly see what has motivated them to think and behave in certain ways throughout their life. When interacting with the therapist, the client may witness how they relate with other people in habitually patterned ways. When journeying in a ceremonial setting, the client may be thrust into *gnosis*, discovering metaphysical truths that transcend doubt. What these various scenarios share is the sudden irruption of unconsciously held mental patterns into explicit awareness, which can free people to make different choices.

This upsurge of the unconscious is not for the faint of heart, however. Most people slowly develop greater self-awareness through psychotherapy, meditation, or other processes of inquiry, circling around their core issues and slowly untangling one knot at a time. Psychedelics are truly the *steep* path up the mountain of knowing oneself. It can be shattering to be confronted with a buried memory of one's own misdeed, or to have an aspect of one's shadow revealed in all its misshapen horror—or, for that matter, to see that one has always been fully loved by God (or the universe) but was unaware. Any of these experiential discoveries can feel like the self is tearing apart, and it requires a lot of stability and ego strength to trust that one can be undone, to have faith that reconstellation can lead to greater flexibility and a more fulfilling life. The therapist's presence and trust in the process can help the client let go and open in this way.

The journeyer may have visions: vivid pictures from the past, symbols of unconscious desires, or undulating geometric patterns that seem to reveal the underlying structure of reality. These mental pictures can be incredibly detailed and evocative. The client may sense the presence of a dissociated aspect of the self, or even the eerie presence of an outside other. Whether we read these encounters as visitations from transpersonal entities, the spirit of the medicine, or coded messages from the unconscious allowing a fuller experiencing of one's depths, it requires a real steadiness of mind in both therapist and client to stay in contact with these phenomena. Encountering a presence that doesn't feel like "me" may be frightening, and yet many journeyers find that these emanations bring healing if approached with openness.

Interoception can help clients access what is usually unconscious. Attending to the spontaneous play of sensations in the body can provide the journeyer with messages that push their process forward. We have found it useful for the therapist to inquire into bodily experiences regularly—not to push away thoughts, feelings, or images but to deepen into the experience of receiving them. We can ask, "What do you feel in your body as you see that image?" Or, "How does that emotion feel in your body?" Sensations may also bring impulses for movement: reaching out for contact, getting up to dance, or even thrashing violently (with adequate support to avoid injury, of course). Wordless vocalizations may come through: moans of grief or pleasure, joyous exclamations, or screams of terror or rage. There's no telling what will come up, and seasoned psychedelic therapists have mostly given up trying to predict how clients will respond. A client behaving uncharacteristically in their journey can be part of the work, as they expand into new ways of being.

PENDULATION

As mentioned, psychedelics will cause clients to unpredictably oscillate between pleasant and unpleasant experiences. This back-and-forth is sometimes confusing for new therapists, who may conceptualize therapy as a dredging up of painful material and attending to it single-mindedly. Or those with a *positive psychology* orientation may be more familiar with fixing attention on things the client feels good about. However, what seems most transformative is a rhythmic shifting between these polarities. As mentioned in Chapter 4, we believe that psychedelics align the body and mind with a natural rhythm between expansion and contraction. This appears to be a critical aspect of the journey's transformative power.

In a recent session, the client swung between polarities in this way: a cascade of potent insights would elicit a wave of grief, with tears flowing freely, and then be punctuated by a little laugh. "Wow, I'm really high," she'd say with a giggle. Then the next wave would come—more revealed truths and gut-wrenching sobs, and then at last more laughter. This is an example of the oscillatory process we're describing.

Peter Levine (1997) recognized the importance of this oscillation long ago, coining the term "pendulation" to describe it. He observed that movement between expansion and contraction was a natural property of organisms—seen in every heartbeat and every breath, as well as in psychological shifts between pain and pleasure—and attending to this became a cornerstone of the SE method. Pendulation is not something the therapist needs to *do* but rather is something that simply happens, and should be highlighted. A swing to one side begets a swing to the other—hence, the image of the pendulum.

Though part of our organismic design, pendulation can get disrupted in trauma and chronic stress. The mental fixations that characterize trauma represent a breakdown of complementarity, a loss of capacity to *hold both*. A central feature of the inner healing intelligence seems to be that it moves between opposites, facilitating healing in an integrative swing between positive and negative. Eventually, this may even lead to that glorious exalted state we could call the undifferentiated, or nondual, where concepts like positive and negative cease to have any meaning—there's just experience, as it is.

It is not the therapist's job to make pendulation happen for the client, but it can be facilitated by highlighting the emergence of *resources*—loci of positive experience—in the client's conscious awareness. It is crucial that the therapist not see pleasure as avoidance or distraction, and attempt to refocus the client's attention on distressing images or thoughts. As the journeyer shifts attention between something scary and something beautiful, or from something sad to something inspiring, the therapist can support and affirm their focus on this new positive element. Levine (2010) recognized the importance of such resources in the integration of trauma, as positive internal experience can potentiate pendulation. The psychedelic therapist should attend to the appearance of a resource in the journey, celebrating the shift from adversity to relief, knowing that it is precisely this movement that mends the mind.

Pendulation also initiates cycles of arousal and settling, restoring the natural rhythm between activation and deactivation in the nervous system. The client need not spend the entirety of a journey in a state of agitation. Ideally, the process is like a shoreline—waves of sympathetic arousal interspersed with calmer, more placid phases. If the journeyer doesn't fixate or try to control things, their experience will naturally cycle between charge and discharge.

The therapist should look out for signs of fixity, of the client being stuck in either a loop of high-charge states or in a stasis where nothing is happening. When someone is stuck in activation, the therapist can intervene with settling, stabilizing, or grounding techniques: encouraging the client to feel their body, take a break from music, orient to the external environment, or receive supportive touch. For the person not experiencing much at all, the therapist might prompt them to remember their intention, move their body, or recall some prior element of the journey that was more active or intense (but perhaps incomplete).

PRESENCE

What is most required of the therapist in these journeys is *presence*. Attending to whatever emerges with open-ended curiosity signals to the journeyer that they are safe and protected. Many educators in the psychedelic space talk about how to develop presence, and people work hard to cultivate this essential capacity.

From our perspective, presence is not something we do—rather, it's something we *stop* doing. Turning away from ruminative, discursive thinking and attending wholeheartedly to the here and now does not require some special new skill set. We simply have to stop getting in our own way. Many meditation teachers describe an inherent wakefulness in the human mind. Attaining enlightenment is not seen as some exalted new mode of being, but rather simply recognizing the realization that is *already there*, and attaining this state is like clouds parting to reveal the brilliant shining sun. Being present—and the capacity to hold space—exist inherently in each of us, awaiting the cessation of extraneous habits of mind that prohibit its emergence.

One way we can help ourselves be present as therapists is to pay close attention to our own embodied experience. The therapist, too, needs to notice when their body becomes overly rigid or collapsed. Muscle fibers, fascial networks, organs, and glands—all of these bodily tissues are incorporated in a bidirectional dance of embodied cognition. Our capacity for presence is tied to the state of our body, and the therapist should regularly direct open and curious attention to their own soma. In order to be present for another we also have to be present to ourselves.

THE INTERPERSONAL FIELD

Attending to our own bodies and supporting our nervous system to be regulated—not too stressed or shut down—can affect the journeyer on a physiological level. Research on *heart rate variability* (HRV), the way the heart and lungs work together, has shown that we implicitly communicate our bodily states to others. Higher HRV is associated with physical health (Jarczok et al., 2022; Tiwari et al., 2021) and psychological wellness (Ramesh et al., 2023). People with higher HRV tend to live longer, healthier, happier lives—up to a certain point, of course, for if HRV is *too* high, that too can signal disease.

Importantly, bodies tend to spontaneously synchronize in terms of HRV measures, *coregulating* to become more resonant. This is probably related to our long evolutionary history as social mammals, where the harmonization of nervous system states would be adaptive for cooperative group life. Our bodies and brains are evolutionarily specialized for coregulation. Although the mechanism for HRV alignment is still unknown, it may be that the heart's electromagnetic signature acts as a beacon to others, inviting them into physiological synchrony. An important finding in at least one study is that the more coherent system usually *wins*—that is, the body with higher HRV will invite the one with lower HRV to match its cadence (Morris, 2010).

All of this research suggests that the therapist is sharing an *interpersonal field* with the journeyer, a co-created atmosphere of physiological and psychological entrainment. Boundaries are still crucial, and differentiation between therapist and client is important for good outcomes. And yet, our bodies are always chugging away in the background, trying to bring us into a synchronous alliance with those around us. Our nervous systems act as transmitters to one another, and what is happening within us matters!

Allowing ourselves to simply be present and available is truly the most important task.

PROTECT THE JOURNEY

Technology can be distracting in the dosing session. Even the best of us occasionally give in to the temptation to check our phones, but best practice is to turn off notifications and minimize intrusions from the outside world. The glow of a screen—for instance, a laptop playing the music—can be a jarring reminder of the day-to-day world the journeyer has left behind. We want the journey space to feel protected, a sanctuary from normalcy that allows the journeyer to roam freely.

We recommend that clients refrain from using their phone or laptop while under the influence. The therapist can maintain a text connection with the client's loved ones—the client may find it meaningful that we've sent a message to someone they care about. These messages should be nonspecific and reassuring. Something along the lines of "They're doing great," will suffice. If supportive messages come back, we can convey these to the client (provided we sense it would be helpful). It can feel incredibly moving for a person on psychedelics to know that their people are rooting for them. However, the therapist must select the appropriate time to relay these messages, not interrupting the client's process or inadvertently making them feel self-conscious. The key principle is to protect the journey, plugging up any energetic "leaks" in the container.

The therapist should consistently check to make sure the journeyer is comfortable. Attending to their physical body is crucial: Make sure they're warm and cozy, and that they have everything they need. Some psychedelic medicines are dehydrating, and the therapist should remind the journeyer to drink water beforehand and to take sips during the journey (it's easy to forget).

Some people will want to talk a lot during their journey, while others may be mostly silent. It's important that the client knows either is okay. It's fine for them to stay internal, as long as they're not getting overwhelmed. Clients who are more talkative may worry that they're being "too much" for the practitioner. Again, people bring their own social habits and their rules about relationships into the journey, and may unconsciously expect us to respond to them the same way others do. In particular, shaming messages the client received in early life may influence their expectations about the psychedelic state. The client may need to be explicitly told, "You're not doing it wrong." We should reassure them that they're understood and supported.

If journeyers do share verbally, the therapist can be their scribe. Quoting the client and taking notes on how the journey develops will provide the session with a written record, which can be a gold mine for the journeyer's later work in the integration process. These hours-long ordeals can be draining, taxing the journeyer's attention and making it difficult to recall everything that happened. The therapist's notes and quotations—perhaps with a time stamp or in relation to songs in the playlist—serves to remind the journeyer of different phases of the session, allowing them to reenter the experience and more deeply assimilate its insights.

TRACKING THE BODY ON PSYCHEDELICS

We need to pay close attention to how the body expresses itself during the journey, keeping a written record of this too. The words and images the client shares are important to notate, but the body narrative is no less important. The therapist can point out these somatic expressions in the moment, helping the journeyer attend to what the body is saying. They can also, however, write down postures, gestures, facial expressions, and other bodily states for later exploration.

Bracing or collapse in the musculature can inhibit emotion and hinder cognitive processing. We might see a client go stiff, or fold into a slackened posture that is crumpled rather than relaxed. Wincing in their face—or curling of their toes—might indicate an unconscious effort to resist the experience. The body may writhe, which could enable the processing of feelings but could also be an attempt to "crawl away" from emotional intensity. When we see avoidance or resistance, we can gently invite the client to let go and open, holding a sense of curiosity for what unfolds.

Another window into the inner experience of a journeyer is the quality of their voice. The larynx and pharynx change in response to internal states, and we can learn much about what's happening based on what we hear. What is the speed of the client's speech? Does it quicken, the words jumbling together? Is it slow and spacey, with overlong gaps between words? What is the pitch? Under stress, our tone of voice rises due to contraction of the voice box. A higher-pitched, tight voice lets us know that the nervous system is amped up, whereas a deeper and more resonant tonality lets us know they've entered a phase of calm.

We can also listen for *prosody* in the voice. This is the sing-song, tonally varying quality of speech used to convey emotion. When the voice is more prosodic it indicates that things are relatively settled and the client is in the phase of social engagement. This biobehavioral state is also associated with higher HRV, the autonomic indicator associated with well-being. When the voice becomes flatter and more unwavering, this cues us that the journeyer is either stressed (if the pitch of the voice is high) or collapsed (if the pitch of the voice is low). If this continues for too long, we might want to invite the journeyer to attend outwardly, allowing access to a more resourced mental state oriented to the here and now. When the voice is more variable, with emotional states communicated through fluctuations in pitch, it lets us know the client's social engagement system has been turned on. We support the process by spontaneously joining them in conversation at these times. Don't be too quick to invite the client back into internal attention (unless you sense they're avoiding something). These experiences of open, compassionate engagement can be very reparative for the client.

It is useful to regularly invite the journeyer into embodied awareness. Images and insights are often immersive, and may cause people to forget that they have a body. For some, the psychedelic state can become quite abstract, uprooting the journeyer from themselves. When clients tune into interoception, feeling sensations in the body instead of just thinking and emoting, it can be very stabilizing and can help them relax and let go. Clients may, at times, feel lost, confused, sense that they need to make an important choice, or "figure things out." It is helpful in these moments to remind them of the soma. Simply say, "Why don't you ask your body?" Or if utilizing music in the work, "Why don't you ask the music?"

The organ of the heart, and the energetic nexus at the center of the rib cage, can be a powerful point of focus during psychedelic work. Though many psychedelics cause an elevated heart rate—distressing for some clients—there is often a sense of warmth and aliveness to be felt in this region of the body. "Ask your heart," is another effective intervention in moments of confusion, either as a metaphor or a prompt to focus on sensations in the chest.

Additionally, we recommend paying close attention to the breath. Respiratory rhythms and patterns can reveal a tremendous amount about what's happening under the surface.

A NONDIRECTIVE APPROACH

Psychedelics release a cascade of vivid images, abnormal thoughts, provocative emotions, and unignorable sensations. In this tangle, it can be difficult to know what to focus on. I [Joshua] have sometimes wondered: "What exactly is *the work*?" As someone holds space for psychedelic sessions, they should trust in the client's inner healing intelligence. Yet, when opening a portal to the unconscious—or, in neuroscience terms, a surge of downstream mental processing—there can be a lot of neurological noise. In other words, not everything that emerges in a journey is worth putting in the spotlight of attention. The brain will at times be deep in a transformative process, at other times adrift on a sea of distorted sensory and cognitive sifting. It can be challenging to recognize which is which.

What we advocate is a nondirective approach. Does this mean that the therapist should attend equally to every element of experience the client reports? No. The therapist must be discerning, and disregard the many "red herrings" that may arise. While it isn't obvious to a neophyte, the experienced psychedelic therapist will be able to intuit which phenomena to reinforce with attention and which to disregard with benign neglect. As this intuition is being developed, though, we suggest inviting the client into body awareness when something emerges that we are unsure about. Grounding attention in this way can dissipate some of the client's fascination with any random neuronal firings that could lead them to distorted meanings.

THE MONSTER IN THE MIRROR

Many paths that arise in the client's consciousness lead to dead ends, and part of the therapist's task is to identify which paths may draw them into greater depths and the possibility of transformation. The ego resists being dismantled, even temporarily, and people can get mired in all kinds of patterns. This archetypal fear of dismantling can symbolically manifest through encounters with demons, monsters, or decay.

When we meet a monster, we can engage it with curiosity and compassion, not attempting to flee or fight against it. However, we don't want to fixate on these encounters, either. One trainee in a psilocybin-assisted therapy program recently reported that his teacher gave the cohort a directive: "If you meet a monster, run toward it and jump into its mouth." This cavalier approach to medicine work is increasingly common, a naive belief that anything psychedelics serve up—no matter how overwhelming—is somehow curative. Clients exposed to such blistering intensity in their journey are simply told to "trust the process." This is a mistake. The principle of non-avoidance—fundamentally trusting and being curious—doesn't mean we should allow for ongoing overwhelm. Psychedelics can expand capacity, but a client's window of tolerance can only handle so much. Exceeding this is rarely, if ever, healing. In fact, habitually gravitating toward greater and greater intensity is often just another avoidance mechanism of the ego.

In *Waking the Tiger,* Peter Levine (1997) invokes the myth of Perseus to describe his approach to healing trauma. The hero Perseus was charged with slaying the gorgon Medusa, a monster with snakes for hair, sharp fangs and claws, and a gaze that turned people to stone. The area around her stronghold was littered with the statues of those who had engaged her head-on. Perseus knew that to look upon Medusa would mean his doom. Instead, he gazed into the mirrored surface of his shield—a gift from the goddess Athena—and slowly approached the monster in the mirror. It was only by beholding the *reflection* of this terrifying form that Perseus could get close enough to vanquish her without becoming frozen in horror.

Trauma is overcome, Levine (1997) argues, not by confronting it head-on but by "working with its reflection, mirrored in our instinctual responses" (p. 65). So it is with the monsters our clients may confront in their journeys. They need not run toward the monster and jump into its mouth. A slow approach from an oblique perspective will bring them close enough to engage it without getting overwhelmed. Many therapists report success with inviting journeyers to meet the monster with compassion, asking it what it needs or what it has come to teach us. We must support clients to notice what arises—whether comforting or scary—without becoming flooded, fixated, or compulsively managing the experience.

It is far easier to *keep* someone out of overwhelm than it is to *get* someone out of overwhelm. We track what is happening in the client's nervous system, noticing their reactions and level of activation, sensing when a client's experience is becoming too much, and intervening *before* they become overwhelmed. We need not shy away from intensity, but we want it to be at a level the client can integrate. Phrases like "I'm right here with you," or a hand on the shoulder, might be all that's needed. We can utilize tools such as weighted blankets, or pillows to squeeze. Again, we don't want clients to avoid confronting the darker aspects of their psyche. What we want is to monitor their level of experiential intensity, heading off these cycles before the point of total overwhelm by introducing resources to make things more bearable.

ENDING THE JOURNEY

At some point, the phase of *return* will feel complete. Sensing that the journeyer has landed back on their feet, we can invite them to contact their support person (or a taxi or rideshare service) to arrange pickup. We shouldn't release someone from our care until we're sure they're back to baseline. It's entirely normal to feel some perceptual or somatic effects of the medicine after coming down, but the journeyer shouldn't still be journeying when they leave.

As mentioned in Chapter 7, it's advisable to preschedule an integration session the day following the journey (or the day after that). The journeyer may struggle with logistics as they come down, so planning in advance is wise. Once their support person arrives, you can send them on their way with contact information for you, the phone numbers of crisis lines in your area, and a plan for what to do in case material from the journey bubbles back up.

CONCLUSION

The psychedelic experience is unlike conventional therapy. It requires practitioners to embrace nonlinearity and discontinuity, to cultivate acceptance and compassion, to be receptive and curious about the journeyer. The therapist joins with the client, avoiding tendencies to either merge or distance. Identifying polarities is key, as well as the naturalistic oscillation between positive and negative experience, arousal and settling. Attending to the body in the journey is the *sine qua non* of psychedelic work—the thing we cannot do without. Arguably, though, the primary task of the therapist is preventing the journey from becoming traumatizing. The utilization of safe, healthy touch can assist with this.

CHAPTER 10

Touch and Psychedelics

Touch is our most social sense.
—TIFFANY FIELDS

Our first touch of water occurs in the womb, as we float in a gentle aquatic embrace. In the warm, amniotic darkness, we are cradled and nourished, enveloped in life-giving waters that protect and sustain us. During the third week of embryonic development, the ectoderm (the outermost layer) and mesoderm (the middle layer, contributing to organ formation) begin laying the foundation for the nervous system and skin. By the fourth week, the neural tube starts developing from the ectoderm, destined to become the central nervous system (the brain and spinal cord). At 6 weeks, the first sensory receptors, such as touch receptors (mechanoreceptors), begin developing in the skin. By the end of the eighth week of gestation, the embryo can respond to touch, exhibiting reflexive movements around the mouth.

The skin, our largest sense organ, blankets the entire body, housing a half million receptors that gather sensory information. As development progresses, touch sensitivity extends to areas like the palms, soles, and parts of the face. These receptors respond to various stimuli: heat, cold, pressure, pain, and pleasure. Our skin develops a tactile language, enabling us to sense and interpret the world around us.

From the moment we are born, human closeness and attachment behaviors are communicated through physical touch. How we are touched becomes a somatic blueprint for healthy relationships. Positive physical touch prepares the nervous system for emotional regulation and physical and intellectual development (Field, 2001). Early caring touch also increases resilience to stress and contributes to a strong immune system.

We don't thrive when we aren't touched. Many decades ago, Spitz (1945) published observations from understaffed orphanages, showing that children who are adequately fed and clothed—but not touched and held—had stunted physical growth and issues with emotion regulation. More recent studies have also shown that institutionalized children who don't receive adequate sensory stimulation show enduring developmental deficits (Ardiel & Rankin, 2010). On the other hand, premature infants who receive gentle massage for 15 minutes, three times a day, appear to gain more weight and have fewer postnatal complications (Field et al., 1986).

A lack of healthy touch may lead to lifelong patterns of avoidance. A study by Lüönd and colleagues (2022) indicates that survivors of childhood maltreatment—whether depressed or not—tend to maintain greater physical distance when interacting with unfamiliar individuals. This preference, which may subtly impact one's sense of social connectedness, reflects the silent impact of early touch deprivation or unhealthy touch.

A coherent inner sense of self develops when humans are affectionately held. This sense of presence involves the comprehension of one's body, attained through precise *proprioceptive* and *vestibular* awareness (proprioception is sensing the body's position and movements while the vestibular sense is related to balance and posture). This facilitates effective emotion-regulation capacities. In other words, we understand and experience ourselves first as a body, through the nurturing touch of a caregiver.

Researchers who study the stress response in rats—whose nervous systems develop much like our own—have demonstrated the importance of mammalian closeness and touch. Some Norway rat caregivers are more attentive than others, licking and grooming their progeny more often. The young of these "high licking and grooming" mothers show a lowered stress response in adulthood (Meaney & Syzf, 2005), increased hippocampal volume (leading to more adaptive learning and memory; Liu et al., 1997), and less vulnerability to cocaine and alcohol dependence (Francis & Kuhar, 2008).

Touch is also regulating for human babies. Physicians now advocate "kangaroo care" (skin-to-skin contact) for low birth weight and preterm infants, as this leads to fewer infections, shorter hospital stays, and drastically lowered mortality rates when compared to conventional neonatal care (Conde-Agudelo & Díaz-Rossello, 2016). Additionally, infants receiving kangaroo care had less circulating cortisol (a hormone involved in the stress response)—and this same physiological profile was seen in their mothers (Cristóbal Cañadas et al., 2022). Mothers offering skin-to-skin contact with their premature infants showed increased oxytocin release (Feldman et al., 2010). Oxytocin, sometimes called the "cuddle hormone," is associated with social bonding, trust, and reduced stress. Oxytocin release regulates physiological functions, such as heart rate (Gutkowska & Jankowski, 2011) and temperature (Zayan et al., 2023).

Touch also regulates the stress response in our bodies. A chronically activated stress response is associated with a range of negative outcomes, including anxiety, depression, addictive behaviors, hypertension, diabetes, inflammation, and heart disease. Healthy, nurturing touch can prevent or alleviate these disease states. Even petting a dog can strengthen the immune system (Charnetski et al., 2004). To feel a true sense of belonging, we need the closeness of others and the comfort of being held. Touch helps us to inhabit our own bodies more fully.

TOUCH AWARENESS

In somatic therapy, we use interpersonal touch when we sense it will be beneficial. This could include imagining physical touch and observing the client's response to that imagery. We help clients distinguish between touch that feels threatening and touch that is welcome and soothing. Ruptures in the relationship, which can damage the therapeutic alliance between therapist and client, may come from physical touch (even when it's meant to be supportive). Most of the time, this happens when the therapist is not clear about their intention and fails to see the impact. Embodied self-awareness and moving mindfully are part of therapeutic touch interventions.

In psychedelic therapy, an emotionally open client may seek physical contact or initiate a hug. This can create vulnerability, especially if the journeyer has a complicated relationship with being touched. A person in an expanded state of consciousness may not always recognize personal boundaries, and may not be able to anticipate how they will later feel about touch. To navigate these situations, therapists must maintain an ethical commitment to clear, professional boundaries, while also ensuring their approach remains compassionate and supportive.

In addition to the complexities of touch during sessions, the client may have a heightened sensitivity to physical proximity and the therapist's body language. Being either too close or too far away can significantly impact the session. Facial expressions, especially when strong emotions are being expressed, become particularly significant in psychedelic therapy. Clients may interpret emotionally ambiguous faces as threatening. Therapists should maintain clearly supportive facial expressions throughout the session.

I [Manuela] was once asked by a psychedelic therapist for consultation. She was integrating therapeutic touch into her practice, and was surprised that a client felt hurt by an intervention meant to be healing. The therapist had offered to gently hold the client's head, rocking it slightly back and forth. This was intended to be a resource as the client reexperienced early familial wounding, and the client reported this *was* a soothing intervention during the preparation session. In the psychedelic dosing session, the client began gripping their head, slightly pulling on their hair, while their neck whipped violently from side to side. The therapist felt compelled to intervene and employed head-holding again. The well-intentioned therapist began rocking the client—but unlike the preparation session, she positioned herself with her legs straddling her client's head. The client stopped their movement. Their breath became shallow, and the body stilled. The therapist took this to mean they had been soothed.

The client reported a markedly different experience during their integration session. They described the therapist's touch as a profound violation, saying it triggered intense fear and a freezing response, as it reminded them of a past trauma involving physical violation. They reported how they had opened their eyes briefly, seeing the therapist's legs positioned close to their body, which had intensified their fear. Seeing this, their body began anticipating potential harm. Additionally, the therapist's rocking motion felt intrusive, out of sync with the client's internal emotional struggle. Consequently, the experience left the client confused, ashamed of their emotions, and torn between their inner knowing and a desire to trust the therapist's authority.

The therapist reassured the client of their good intentions and highlighted their expertise in therapeutic touch. However, despite these efforts, a rupture had occurred and was not repaired. The client did not return; trust had been irreparably damaged, and the therapist was puzzled about what had gone wrong. The therapist missed an opportunity to inquire empathetically into the client's discomfort without defensiveness, which could have validated and empowered the client. Additionally, the therapist missed the opportunity to explore her own defensiveness.

In expanded states, the body perceives sensations and emotions differently. While touch can offer support, it also has the potential to feel violating and triggering, casting the journeyer back into memories of prior trauma. Effective touch practice involves adhering to agreements and guidelines, while also remaining keenly observant of the client's responses. This balance requires both artistry and professional humility—we can't simply follow a predetermined protocol.

GENERAL GUIDELINES ON THERAPEUTIC RELATIONAL TOUCH

Adhering to guidelines is essential when employing touch. Therapists must approach physical contact with careful consideration, thorough training, and heightened awareness.

As therapists, we should consider adopting the following ethical guidelines:

- Wherever possible, train in the use of ethical and safe touch.

- Know your profession's legal and ethical guidelines and your scope of practice.
- Never touch a client without their consent.
- Keep your original touch agreements from the preparation session.
- Sexual or romantic contact is never therapeutic between a therapist and a client.
- No full-body contact, such as cuddling.
- Safe touch is clean, nonthreatening touch. If you have any hesitation or doubts about the clinical value of touch, don't do it.
- Discuss and empower the client to confidently decline physical contact and assertively say no when necessary.
- Do not assume that touch-based interventions are always helpful for clients.
- Notice the body. If you ask for consent and the client hesitates, consider not touching. If the client says "Yes" but then the body contracts (or goes cold) when we touch, remove the contact and explore the person's response.

THE FOUR TYPES OF TOUCH

All touch interventions must be performed with the utmost care. The four types of touch described below will be employed at different times, depending on the therapist's intention. For example, the therapist might want to direct the client's attention to a specific area of their body—or may want to help the client feel more stable.

> *Reassuring touch*: This type of touch is calm, steady, and caring. Reassuring touch helps the client befriend a fear or cope with a moment of disorientation. It assures the cli-

ent they can let go and trust their experience. For example, we may offer support by gently holding their hand or placing a hand on their tensed shoulder. You might add soothing words, or sing a gentle song, offering assurances to the client when they're feeling vulnerable. Reassuring touch generally evokes a sense of being *held*, a reminder that the therapist is an ally in the experience.

Hands-on touch: This refers to touch used to guide the client's attention to a specific body area. This approach employs distinct therapeutic objectives tailored to the client's individual needs and circumstances. For example, placing a hand on the client's arm or feet directs their focus there, potentially addressing blockages or highlighting areas that are offline. Additionally, this kind of touch can assist the client in discovering inner resources and finding alignment or relaxation in particular areas of the body. This touch encourages clients to remain present with their experience and enhances their therapeutic journey. It is essential to observe changes in the client's breath, such as shifts in the rhythm or depth of respiration, which provides valuable insight into their emotional and physiological state.

Containing touch: When a client is restless, thrashing, or in significant discomfort, touch is used to contain intense energy and ensure physical safety. At times, the client will need to feel a boundary—and there may also be moments when we need to insist on physically supporting the journeyer (please see *non-negotiable touch* below). People on psychedelics sometimes feel a powerful charge coursing through them, and their bodies may start to move all on their own. Both of these things could be disturbing or scary. The therapist's confident application of physical support can make all the difference.

Facilitating touch: This touch *facilitates* sensorimotor processing when the client is having trouble expressing something (e.g., a stuck emotion, or a dynamic physical movement). Highly energetic movements might need physical support to be completed. Sometimes these movements are tied to memories, perhaps the completion of self-protective responses unable to be enacted at the time of a trauma. Or they can be purely somatic, without a narrative. Muscle tension can be alleviated by applying pressure while the client actively resists, creating an isometric contraction. During this process, the muscle remains contracted as it resists the pressure, helping to complete motor patterns and empowering clients. This technique can be particularly useful for addressing physical tensions stuck in the body. However, it is a sensitive and potentially quite provocative approach, requiring proper touch training to apply ethically. It must always be performed with careful clinical judgment while respecting any dissent or verbal objections from the client. Once this strong energetic movement is released, inviting the client to rest is important. Encourage them to mindfully attend to their breath and body, promoting relaxation and integration.

GAIN CONSENT TO TOUCH

In preparing for psychedelic-assisted therapy, it is crucial to discuss the potential use of touch in detail. This includes informing the client about ethical touch guidelines and discussing the types of touch that may be utilized when they consent to it. This proactive approach helps establish clear boundaries and promotes a therapeutic environment that prioritizes the client's comfort and safety.

Inform the client that touch in psychedelic therapy differs from massage. It is not intended to relieve physical pain or manipulate physical tissue; instead, the role of touch is to support the therapeutic process. Touch may involve hand-holding, adjusting body posture for comfort with pillows and blankets, providing support during moments of fear, gently containing agitation, and offering soothing contact during moments of distress. Or we might need to offer support during a trip to the bathroom. Again, emphasize that therapeutic touch strictly excludes any form of sexual or romantic touch. There may be times when the therapist's touch is required, which we call non-negotiable touch. To be clear: preventing injury is the only time when touch is non-negotiable. For example, if the client could potentially injure themselves with physical expression, or fall when standing or moving, our role as protector becomes paramount. We do whatever is necessary to keep the person from any physical harm while in the expanded state, even if this contact feels unwelcome in the moment. Using pillows or props can be helpful.

Invite a conversation about the client's history and what associations they might have with touch. Learn what touch means to the client, inquiring into any culturally based sensitivities there could be. You might ask, "What kind of touch norms were in your family and culture? What past experiences with touch have been positive or negative? What kind of touch are you afraid of?" Find out about any physical violations or trauma related to touch. If a client has experienced relational, physical, or sexual abuse or assault, it is crucial to use extra caution. Discuss the use of touch and the boundaries surrounding it, conducting a thorough touch inventory and assessment.

Exercise: Exploring Consent

This preparatory exercise is useful when considering touch in psychedelic therapy. Discuss the exercise with your client beforehand, encouraging them to practice saying "No" to touch and observing any internal conflicts that arise. Common experiences include wanting to say "No"—but not wanting to disappoint the therapist, feeling conflicted about wanting and not wanting touch simultaneously, or being afraid of violation. As the therapist, frame this inquiry as a mindful exploration, focusing on what is associated with touch in a therapeutic setting. Importantly, no physical touch will occur during this exercise; the goal is to observe the client's internal reactions to the offer of touch. Together, discuss and understand these reactions and establish clear agreements that will be respected in psychedelic therapy sessions.

In this exercise, we explore three different scenarios to study the impact of touch. After each scenario, pause to discuss and analyze what occurred before moving on to the next step.

SCENARIO 1: THERAPIST OFFERS TOUCH

Therapist's offer:
- Example: "I would like to offer to hold your hand right now."

Client's response:
- Notice your immediate response and bodily sensations. Are you calm, relaxed, tense, confused, or something else?

    Report back to the therapist what you felt after being offered touch.

SCENARIO 2: CLIENT ASKS FOR TOUCH

Client's request:
- Example: "Can you hold my hand?"

Client's response:
- Observe what it feels like to ask for touch and what emotions or thoughts are evoked. Do you feel conflicted? Is this okay for you? Reflect on your experience.

SCENARIO 3: THERAPIST OFFERS TOUCH AND CLIENT SAYS "NO"

Therapist's offer:
- Example: "I will hold your hand now, just as we discussed."

Client's response:
- Focus on your inner response to the offer, particularly if you feel any sense of hesitation or even a subtle cringe. Where do you feel this? Is there any conflict about expressing it?

Practice expressing "No":
- Verbal examples: "No," "Please don't," "I actually don't want that," and so on.
  Nonverbal examples: Shake your head, put up a hand in a "Stop" gesture, pull your hand into your body, or turn your body away.
  Study this experience and see what arises as you set the boundary.

After each scenario, discuss what comes up together. You can also reflect together on what these experiences mean for your upcoming psychedelic session. Consider the following:

- What is your comfort level with touch?
- What does touch mean to you?
- Do you want to include therapeutic touch?
- What would help you to say "No"?

By thoroughly exploring and discussing these scenarios, you and your therapist can better understand and establish clear, respectful boundaries regarding touch in your psychedelic therapy sessions.

ETHICAL ISSUES IN THE USE OF TOUCH

Though the human organism seems designed to receive healthy touch as pleasant, a person's history may condition them to feel aversion to contact. Deciding not to receive touch must be given as a legitimate option. During the preparation phase, the therapist inquires into which forms of touch the client finds most supportive—or if they prefer to decline touch. This ensures our approach will provide the greatest therapeutic benefit.

Sometimes a client will decline touch in the preparation session but then request it when they're high, which raises a complex ethical question. Some would say that it is imperative that the therapist honor the original agreement—a psychedelically altered person has diminished capacities, after all. This principled stance protects the client from intimacy that might later be seen as a violation. At the same time, the therapist might struggle with the ethics of denying the journeyer the healing balm of contact in their moment of need. Clear agreements beforehand are important. We suggest that the therapist default to holding the boundary the client originally set for themselves when sober; at times, though, a renegotiation of this agreement may feel absolutely necessary to the journeyer.

At other times, a client who said they will want touch in their journey during preparation—and who assents to touch when asked—discovers that it feels off in some way when they receive it. It can be difficult to speak up about this, particularly when in an altered state. Some therapists have the client practice declining touch during preparation sessions. For instance, the therapist might lay a hand on the client's forearm and—whether or not the touch is experienced as negative—invite the client to say "No," and to feel what it's like when the therapist respects this boundary by withdrawing their hand. This can create a template for response during the dosing session, when it can sometimes be difficult to connect with a clear intention about being touched.

We must also abide by the guidelines of our licensure. Some psychotherapists are constrained by their licensing boards in terms of what kinds of physical contact are allowable. In places where psychedelic work is legal, certain types of touch may be forbidden in dosing sessions. Practitioners operating in such aboveground contexts should consult the current regulations before proceeding.

Discuss any nonverbal cues you need to know about that would indicate a need for touch. For example, if the client reaches a hand toward you during the session, is that a nonverbal request for contact? Likewise, ask if they have any objections to touch. Discuss the cues for consent to touch and emphasize that this will always be respected. Be specific and clear. The more you learn and discuss, the more comfortable the client will be when you offer touch.

Case Study: Marcus

In our intake, Marcus shared with me [Manuela] that while he generally welcomed touch, there had been times when he'd felt aversive to it. He was conflicted about rejecting touch, worried that he would offend other people—or that if he refused, the other person would abandon him.

When I asked him how, during his ketamine journey, he would recognize not wanting to be touched by me, he replied that he would feel an internal "No." He described one indicator of his discomfort as a sensation of withdrawing internally, as though he were pulling away from the contact.

I knew I needed to learn more about his dilemma. Because this was a core issue, he agreed that negotiating touch would likely be important in the session. I asked him how I could learn more about this internal "No." He reported that if he was conflicted inside about touch, he would "go cold," and suggested this could be a cue for me to release contact.

In the psychedelic session, when I held Marcus's hand, his grip turned limp and his hand became chilly, as if he was ready to end a handshake. My sense was that I was contacting someone who no longer wanted to meet my hand. Remembering that this was his cue, I asked permission to slowly withdraw my hand and gently placed his hand to his chest.

In the integration session, he expressed gratitude that I was attentive to his needs. It was a pivotal moment: He had asked for touch when he wanted it, and he got it—but when his needs changed, I was attuned to the shifting landscape of his inner experience. He felt me listening in that moment, capable of noticing a subtle shift. Unlike his typical ambivalent attachment experiences, he could navigate his complex emotions while feeling supported—without fearing the loss of connection. This newfound experience of being deeply listened to on a somatic level facilitated a transformation in Marcus's relational patterns.

ATTUNE TO NONVERBAL CONSENT AND DISSENT CUES

Consenting to touch isn't just about signing a form in the preparation session. Once preliminary consent is established, ongoing attention to the evolving experience in the present moment is required. Giving consent to touch once does not imply consent forever; this work necessitates continual listening and respect for shifting needs and boundaries. Check your assumptions, and don't utilize touch unless *you* feel comfortable with it. Here are some questions you can ask yourself:

- How does the client respond to the touch you are giving?
- What are you tracking visually in the client's body as you provide touch?
- What are you noticing in your body as you provide touch? Do you feel like you're being received?
- Is there tension or bracing as you touch (in yourself *or* the client)?
- Or is there a deepening of breath or vocalizations of ease?
- Are there any subtle cues that suggest a "No"?
- Can you take care of *your* needs as you provide the touch?

Try This: Tracking the Inner "No"

Recall a moment when someone touched you without your consent. Ensure it's not a traumatic memory but a casual instance, such as someone accidentally touching your arm or encroaching too closely, making you uncomfortable. The purpose is to study how your body immediately recognized and felt a somatic "*No.*"

Close your eyes and notice how that felt in your body. What did you observe? Were you startled? Was there an impulse to withdraw or brace yourself? How did your breathing change in that moment? What do you remember about your body's response at that time? As you bring this memory to mind now, what sensations or reactions do you notice in your body?

ASSESS YOUR ROLE

Reflecting on your personal history and biases is essential. Question your motivations: Why do think touch would be helpful now? Clarify your intentions and assessments carefully. Monitor your comfort level closely to avoid overstepping your own boundaries, as clients can sense discomfort during the psychedelic journey.

Some therapists might touch to ease their discomfort with emotional intensity—which can be unconscious. In this case, recognizing the self-serving quality of the intervention is important, and with this realization they can quickly refocus on the client's needs rather than their own. Check in with yourself if you feel anxious, and work with your own activation, orienting to the external environment to settle or practicing grounding exercises.

Touching a client can evoke various reactions, such as crying, shaking, deep breath releases, and vocalizations. Observe what happens in your body as you witness these reactions. When somatic tensions are released, relational intimacy and relief often follow. Pay attention to your response in these moments. Your self-awareness and emotional regulation are crucial to maintaining a safe and supportive environment for the client.

SELF-TOUCH

Self-touch can be an effective intervention, and we recommend teaching your client strategies for self-touch during the preparation session(s). When guiding the client in using self-touch, sensitivity to their cultural norms is essential. Some clients may feel uncomfortable with self-touch, so be attentive to what works for them and never insist on touch of any kind.

Introducing self-touch practices can evoke deeper layers of memories, emotions, and unresolved trauma. Practicing these exercises in the preparation phase helps clients recognize touch as a valuable tool. Familiarizing clients with self-touch and its ability to calm the nervous system fosters inner somatic resources.

Discuss what kinds of self-touch are helpful and calming, such as placing a hand on the chest and/or belly to regulate breathing. Teach simple self-touch exercises that can be remembered during psychedelic therapy. Encourage them to practice self-touch as homework. By doing this, clients can develop a deeper connection with their bodies, learn to self-regulate, and create a sense of safety and grounding that can be beneficial during their therapeutic journey.

Try This: Skin-to-Skin Listening

This straightforward yet impactful exercise introduces clients to the potency of self-touch as a tool for regulation, grounding, and connecting with their soma. Here's a suggested script for conducting this exercise in the preparation phase with your client.

Use your nondominant hand and mindfully approach a part of your body where the skin is exposed, such as a forearm or the top of your chest.

Don't perform any touch yet; slowly approach this area, being mindful of your breath. Slow down and open your senses.

Hover your hand over the spot. Imagine the inside of your palm has sensitive receptors. Sense the skin area before you touch the actual body. Listen deeply to what you're receiving underneath your hand right now.

Then, place your palm on the skin. What are you sensing from your palm in the skin area?

Take a few slow breaths and let the inner receptors of your hands receive.

Now, switch your focus. Let the skin area touch your inner palm. Imagine that your skin is receiving and sensing the quality of touch from your hand. What do you notice now?

USE OF TOUCH IN THE PREPARATION PHASE

In all three phases of psychedelic therapy, we can apply ethical therapeutic touch in trauma-informed ways. In the preparation phase, learn about somatic markers and associations with touch arising from the client's history. Give the client time to consider their relationship to touch and discern what is appropriate and what is not.

The preparation phase is a pivotal stage for learning, where clients can uncover protective mechanisms. For instance, a client who consistently overworks—or appears dissociated and stoic—may give the impression of being healthy and in control. However, chronic stress and defensiveness are often beneath this behavior. Mindful explorations of somatic responses to touch can help uncover what's beneath compensatory strategies. Feelings of danger, overwhelm, confusion, chaos, and collapsed willpower can be explored.

USE OF TOUCH IN THE JOURNEY PHASE

Orienting Clients to Touch

After gaining consent, it's helpful to orient your client to touch before it comes. Orienting to touch means stating clearly what you will be doing at any given moment. This lowers anticipatory anxiety about what will happen and sets expectations about the kind of contact that will be made. The client will understand what to expect and have time to decline if they want.

In a psychedelic session, there might be a moment when you need to adjust the environment or sit close to the client for comfort. Here is how you can verbalize your approach to touching (usually prefaced with invitational language asking for permission, such as "Would it be OK with you if . . . "):

> "I am going to adjust your pillow, so you are more comfortable."
> "I'm going to come closer and hold your hand."
> "I am moving so I can support you better."
> "I will move back now. "
> "I'm about to put my hand on your shoulder."

Orienting the client to your proximity and touch communicates care, reassuring the journeyer that they can relax, not be hypervigilant, but still maintain an awareness of boundaries (even in an altered state).

When Touch Is Not Possible

Using props can be helpful when physical touch is not possible. For example, you can use a weighted blanket to create a feeling of holding, useful when the client does not want contact but still wants to feel held or contained.

Placing firm pillows behind a head or back can also provide a sense of being supported and held—and we can also remind clients of the potential resource of self-touch.

Try This: Listening Self-Touch

Sit quietly and become aware of your breath. Rest your hands in your lap comfortably, relaxing your body. Close your eyes, placing your attention inward. Allow yourself to slow down, sensing your body at the skin level. Imagine that your skin is breathing with the rhythm of your inhalation and exhalation, subtly expanding and contracting. Now, scan your body from head to toe, seeing if there is an area of the body that feels like it wants contact. Maybe you notice a body part that feels tense, or one that is numb. Slowly place one of your hands on that area of the body. Notice what it's like to have your hand resting there, seeing what other sensations arise and if there is any change to your respiration. Now, begin to "listen" with your hand, sensing what your palm or fingertips are receiving from this part of the body. What do you notice? What is this part of your body asking for, or communicating? And what changes as you pay attention? You can remove your hand, notice any effect, and then return it. Look for some kind of shift, either in the part of the body you're touching, in your breath, in your sense of presence, or even fluctuations in your body temperature. Next, open your attention again, seeing if there's a different area of your body that would like to receive touch. If there is, bring your hand there. It could be your other hand, keeping your first hand where it is, or you can move from one place to the other and see what happens. Rest in this way for a few breaths, being curious if other shifts occur. You can make this inquiry repeatedly, contacting other parts of the body. When you feel done, remove your hand(s) and simply rest, opening your awareness to sense the body as a whole. What is different?

Tracking Cues

Observe bodily indicators that convey the touch is being received positively. Look for a hand that reaches out to you, or that responds with a squeeze to hand-holding. Notice if hands-on touch to the shoulders is followed by a release of breath, a softening, a sigh, or a vocalization, all of which can indicate receptivity. Track for signs such as the easing of muscle tension, breath deepening or slowing down, and skin color darkening with increased blood flow. These indicators can help you understand whether the touch is well received and can guide your approach.

When touch is well received, clients may mutter a soft "Thank you," or shed gentle tears of gratitude. A cool hand that gradually warms to the touch can indicate a transition out of "freeze." Whole-body trembling can occur as defensive body armor eases. Subtle, tiny movement impulses might emerge, promoting greater embodiment. Track all of these body indicators of integration; they will become a road map to understanding the client's inner somatic landscape.

Intense Energy Release

Touch evokes many dimensions of memory. Powerful traumatic memories can arise quickly and be surprising. Sensorimotor impulses related to survival, such as fight, flight, and freeze responses, can surface in response to feeling threatened. Experiences of embodied awakening—such as unfreezing or strong energetic discharges—can be expressed physically.

The energy released in the body can lead to an expansion of consciousness, such as the awakening of a vital life force known as *kundalini*. *Kundalini*, in the Hindu tradition, is a spiritual energy coiled at the base of the spine. During mystical experiences, the body can move into uncontrollable shaking, jerky sharp movements, fast breathing, hyperventilation, and intense vibrational sensations. Vivid visual imagery can bring sudden and unpredictable behaviors, such as laughing out loud, crying, vocalizing, and sounding. These intense experiences are often associated with enduring positive shifts in creativity, presence, and spontaneity. Many people discover they've been unconsciously thwarting the emergence of their life force.

During intense emotional moments, clients may experience a variety of physical symptoms. Some of these complaints might include feeling somatic pains, headaches, and nausea. Temperature fluctuations—feeling alternately hot and cold—are also common. In these moments, we might see clients holding parts of their body for self-comfort.

Strong emotional charge might cause movements: pressing the entire body against the bed, or curling into a tight, embryonic position. Clients may have embodied memories of traumatic birth moments, out-of-body or near-death experiences, and archetypal or past-life experiences. All of these situations may be aided by touch, to ground the person in the here and now and remind them we are there, containing their experience. Also, knowing when to step back and allow the process to unfold, trusting the client's inner healer, is essential.

USE OF TOUCH IN THE INTEGRATION PHASE

In integration sessions, review your preparatory agreements about touch and revisit the moments of physical touch from the journey, inquiring into the client's feelings. Be open and receptive to feedback on whether the touch was welcome. If the client expresses discomfort or doubt, shift into curious listening, remaining undefended and open. Avoid justifying why you used touch. This is a critical area in which relational injury can occur, potentially leading to feelings of shame, being shut down, or being misunderstood, resulting in a therapeutic rupture. Check if repair is needed, perhaps in the form of an unqualified apology.

If self-touch or relational touch during the session was powerful, mindfully explore its healing effects in the integration session(s). For example, you might say, "So, you liked it when you touched your heart. At that moment, it seemed that you were connected to a deeper mystery. Was that your experience? As you remember that, what does it evoke for you now?" Clients will remember sensations related to touch in their journey more vividly when the actual touch and gesture is repeated. The body retains the memory of that sacred moment; by repeating it, the client can make the meaning conscious. Somatic integration allows experiences to be accessed again in the present moment, anchored in an ordinary state of consciousness and integrated. Memories of touch can bridge the mystical state and everyday life, facilitating new insights and meanings. The Touch Outcomes Measurement Inventory (TOMI), developed for MDMA-AT, could be a helpful tool for assessing the impact of touch interventions (Luoma, 2023).

CONCLUSION

When used wisely in psychedelic therapy, touch can powerfully support healing in the client's journey. Introducing touch in the preparation phase—as well as thoroughly debriefing touch interventions in the integration phase—helps minimize potential harm. Understanding the client's preferences around touch can ease discomfort for both the journeyer and therapist. Making clear agreements before the session is crucial. Ethics experts recommend written agreements, encouraging clients to reflect, in writing, on how they feel about touch as well as documenting agreements with the therapist (Taylor, 2017). These agreements could include when and how the therapist may touch the client during the session as well as the client's acknowledgment that the therapist may have to violate the agreement to prevent injury to the client. For instance, even if the client has indicated they don't want to be touched, the therapist may have to help steady them as they go to the restroom. Or, they may need to contain the client if a sudden impulse to thrash could create bodily harm. These agreements should be part of the written consent form, or forms. The more open and detailed your conversations are, the cleaner your therapeutic container will be.

CHECKLIST: THE FOUR Rs

This simple four-step process reminds therapists of the key stages in offering healthy therapeutic touch:

- ☐ Request
  - Discuss the possible benefits of touch, emphasizing that it is never required.
  - Clearly outline permitted types of touch (e.g., holding hands, shoulder contact) and any restrictions.
  - Request their explicit verbal (and/or written) consent to be touched (or to not be).
- ☐ Review
  - Before each session, review the client's consent for

therapeutic touch, ensuring it aligns with their established boundaries and agreements.
- ○ Reinforce that clients can decline touch anytime without needing to justify their decision.
- ○ Discuss nonverbal cues—such as withdrawing a hand—as possible signals of withdrawing consent.

☐ Renew
- ○ Obtain renewed consent for touch before making contact, regardless of past agreements.
- ○ Remind clients that the touch is for their benefit. Follow up to see how they are experiencing it, confirming that it is helpful.

☐ Revoke
- ○ Emphasize that clients can revoke consent for touch at any moment.
- ○ Create a permissive environment in which clients feel comfortable communicating their needs, without any fear of upsetting their therapist.

CHAPTER 11

Trauma and Psychedelics

*I will walk with you through the darkness,
as you remember your light.*
—SHEREE BLISS TILSLEY

Trauma profoundly disconnects people from their bodies and everyday lives. As a client once described it: "I feel like I'm looking through a foggy glass at a world I should belong to . . . but I don't know how to reach it." Trauma survivors often grapple with disrupted mental and physical health, and strained relationships with family and friends. They may withdraw socially and struggle with emotional volatility. Intrusive memories, nightmares, sleep disturbance, negative thinking, and unexplained physical ailments may also plague them.

Thankfully, psychedelics have shown promise in clinical studies for people with treatment-resistant PTSD (Krediet et al., 2020; Mithoefer et al., 2011). Psychedelic therapies can help address trauma at its root, offering significant relief from debilitating symptoms. They also facilitate a search for meaning and spiritual connection—ushering in positive effects that may endure for months, or even years.

Both psychedelic and somatic therapies are effective treatments for trauma. Combining them under the care of a skilled practitioner can create synergistic effects, making them even more effective.

THE TRAUMA CONTINUUM

The American Psychological Association (2023) has surveyed psychologists, gathering evidence that a wide variety of traumas are on the rise. According to the National Center for PTSD (2023), PTSD affects around 13 million adults in the United States alone. Unfortunately, conventional psychiatric drugs have a limited effect in treating this complex disorder (Zaretsky et al., 2024).

Trauma exists on a continuum, manifesting in various forms, each with a unique impact:

> *Developmental trauma* disrupts a child's growth and emotional development, whereas *attachment trauma* affects relational bonding and influences future relationship patterns.
> *Shock trauma* results from sudden, atypical events, such as accidents, assaults, and combat. Sexual violence often leaves survivors with profound fears about their bodies and intimate relationships. Hearing about the trauma of another person—especially when it is graphic or especially horrifying—can leave a person with *secondary trauma.*
> *Collective traumas*—including pandemics, terrorism, natural disasters, and community violence—leave lasting scars on entire populations, expressed via symptoms in individuals.
> *Intergenerational trauma* is when one's ancestors pass down unprocessed trauma, encoded into our DNA and/or transmitted through behavior. This can be characterized by chronic pathologies passed down through fam-

ilies: domestic violence, addiction, suicide, and other destructive behaviors.

Trauma therapists and psychedelic therapists often experience burnout and compassion fatigue from their exposure to clients' trauma. Also, existential dread—pervasive fear and distress about environmental degradation, natural disasters, and the uncertain future of our planet—can contribute to a sense of helplessness, leaving people depressed or anxious.

THE WISDOM OF TRAUMA

Physician and addiction expert Gabor Maté (2024) describes trauma as an "invisible force that shapes our lives" (para. 1). As psychological trauma influences our cognitive and emotional frameworks, it determines things like our relationships and career choices. While trauma often involves a narrowing of perspective (what some have called "tunnel vision"), the study of posttraumatic growth has clarified that this invisible force can also improve our lives if overwhelming experiences can be metabolized and a broader perspective gained.

Psychedelic therapy can help broaden one's perspective, fostering a profound sense of acceptance. A study by Sweeney et al. (2022) at Johns Hopkins University found that both near-death experiences and psychedelic experiences altered people's attitudes toward life. Participants reported a reduced fear of death and a more positive outlook following these transformative experiences. Notably, psychedelics often include a spiritual dimension. Two thirds of volunteers in one study rated their psilocybin session as one of their life's top five spiritual experiences (Griffiths et al., 2006).

One client described a profound encounter with a "loving universe," a "godlike presence," that significantly contributed to their healing process. This experience allowed them to contextualize past traumas within a larger, sacred framework, resulting in shifts in perception and internalized beliefs. They subsequently reported feeling more warmly toward themselves. We've seen how somatically informed psychedelic therapy often improves self-acceptance and self-compassion.

TRAUMA HEALING WITH MDMA

MDMA has shown great promise in treating trauma. MDMA seems to temporarily downregulate fear-processing centers in the brain, facilitating the reprocessing of traumatic memories without the associated [overwhelming] emotions. MDMA enables individuals to access and integrate details of trauma that may have been desperately avoided—or even banished from memory completely.

Research trials conducted by MAPS have demonstrated that providing MDMA-assisted psychotherapy is an effective treatment for PTSD (Mithoefer et al., 2011), including for military veterans with treatment-resistant cases (Mithoefer et al., 2018). Mitchell et al. (2021) found that 67% of participants in their treatment group—receiving MDMA combined with psychotherapy—no longer met the criteria for PTSD. Fully 88% of this cohort experienced a significant reduction in symptoms, compared to 32% in the placebo group.

MDMA increases emotional openness, heightens compassion, enhances social engagement, and allows for the disclosure of sensitive psychological material, making it particularly effective in treating trauma. MDMA works on neurotransmitter receptors in serotonergic and dopaminergic pathways, while also elevating oxytocin levels—which increases empathy and self-compassion. This neurobiological state creates the ideal conditions for processing traumatic events and recovering from PTSD.

Case Study: Jared

Jared was a skilled scout sniper renowned for his expertise in reconnaissance and marksmanship. He served 8 years in the army before a profound change in his personality began impacting his life.

Unfortunately, the traits that made him so successful on missions made it difficult to connect with loved ones at home. Jared became emotionally distant and increasingly isolated from friends and family. Haunted by memories of killing people in the line of duty, he lay awake at night replaying these events. Jared grappled with guilt and shame about harming innocent bystanders, betraying his religious values. He had difficulty falling asleep, and experienced frequent nightmares when he did.

Despite seeking professional help, he had found little relief. In desperation, he began to self-medicate with alcohol and cannabis. He was eventually discharged from the army.

By the time I [Manuela] met Jared, he had undergone several underground MDMA and psilocybin sessions. He reported some benefit from these journeys, though they had not restored his sense of self-worth or fully resolved his symptoms. So, he sought out somatic trauma therapy.

After several sessions of building rapport, introducing essential somatic resources and regulation techniques, we had a breakthrough. Jared had described a sensation that felt like a switch inside him had flipped. He had experienced this before on missions, and also during his journeys—his sniper-self coming online, present for the heat of battle but emotionally absent.

For the first time I observed Jared's stillness, his eyes narrowing as if zeroing in on a target. His lips pursed, jaw tensing, his breath shallow and even.

A chill ran through me as I watched him assume this deadly focus. I took a slow, deliberate breath, allowing my body to mirror his.

A part of him seemed to make way for the sniper to take control.

I asked, "Who is here right now?"

"My soldier," Jared said, fixing a cool, detached gaze on me.

We sat in silence, the fear rising within me. I softened my face, smoothed my voice. "And who has to leave for the soldier to be here?"

His jaw tightened, face flushed with emotion, but he said nothing.

"This must be exhausting, huh?" I said, holding his gaze.

Jared began to cry. "I was so young . . . ," he whispered. "I was *so young*."

I felt a strong sense of connection with him, and my fear

ebbed away. I said emphatically, "Of course you were. I'm so sorry you had to experience that horror, and at such a young age. How unfair..."

Jared shared that he felt a part of him die during his military training. I mourned this death with him, acknowledging and normalizing his shame, pain, and guilt. He told me that he just wanted compassion, and that despite forgiving himself during his journeys he'd never received forgiveness from anyone else. Suddenly, his younger self emerged: vulnerable, scared, and conflicted.

Through guided imagery, we walked this idealistic 18-year-old home. I asked if we could hold the young man together. Jared cradled his midsection, his chest heaving with sobs. In that moment, I felt like a universal mother, present to his pain, witnessing his bravery, safeguarding his vulnerability. This was the integration he needed—to be seen and understood in his most vulnerable state—without judgment from his soldier persona. Jared had finally come home.

I feel certain that Jared's experiences with MDMA made this integration possible, but also recognize that he needed a skilled relational therapist to facilitate this final homecoming, integrating his trauma and moral injury. The effects of a psychedelic journey often linger, making later somatic sessions more impactful.

EMPATHY AND BURNOUT IN THE TRAUMA THERAPIST

Victims of severe trauma often resist distressing memories and intense emotions. Such avoidance requires substantial mental effort, draining the client's energy. This presents a formidable challenge in conventional therapy.

Therapists, despite their best efforts, may inadvertently convey feelings of frustration in response to this resistance. This frustration, unfortunately, might just reinforce the client's pessimistic view of their recovery prospects.

Empathy and compassion are vital to the therapeutic process. Over time, though, empathic responses to traumatized clients can deplete the therapist's own emotional reserves. One study has demonstrated the significant role of *vicarious trauma*—a secondary effect in which hearing another person's trauma creates symptoms in the listener—on clinician burnout (Kounenou et al., 2023). Burnout makes it difficult, or impossible, to maintain the therapeutic presence necessary for effective treatment.

TRAUMA AND THE AUTONOMIC NERVOUS SYSTEM

Trauma seems to be stored in the brainstem, expressed as dysregulation in the *autonomic nervous system* (ANS). The ANS operates on an unconscious level, regulating heart rate, respiration, digestion, pupillary response, sexual arousal, and a host of other physiological variables. It consists of two branches: the sympathetic and parasympathetic nervous systems. The sympathetic is excitatory, involved in the stress response, while the parasympathetic is inhibitory, responsible for settling. Animals first evolved a parasympathetic system, facilitating the response biologists call *energy conservation*. This biobehavioral state can immobilize us when faced with inescapable threat. This self-protective sequence, known as the "freeze" response, ensured that our animal forebears could survive by becoming very still, feigning death and thereby avoiding predation.

Peter Levine (1997) posits that the fundamental ingredient of trauma is the experience of helplessness in the presence of a threat. He emphasizes that when individuals are confronted with overwhelming situations, feeling powerless to escape or repel an invader, it can lead to lasting psychological effects. This underscores the importance of addressing feelings of helplessness in trauma recovery; restoring a sense of agency is crucial for healing. In an event seen as life-threatening, our organism knows that one of the smartest things we can do—especially if our "fight-or-flight" response hasn't worked—is to surrender. Even though this surrender may have allowed a person to survive, it may represent one of the worst moments of a person's life, and feel like failure. It's essential, then, to acknowledge that a psychedelic therapist's directive to "let go" or "surrender" may feel threatening to traumatized clients. Encouraging these clients to "trust the process" may clash with their deep-seated need to avoid vulnerability, a response shaped by past experiences.

I [Manuela] worked with a client who had PTSD from childhood abuse in a spiritual cult and had previously sought healing through a group psychedelic journey. During the preparation phase, the guide informed her that surrendering was a vital part of the process. Although she agreed on a conceptual level and was enthusiastic about the work, the term "surrender" triggered a response in her. In her journey, she relived a memory of being locked in a dark room as a child. The guide's instruction to surrender felt like a command from her abusers, causing her to hyperventilate with fear.

Had the guide instead offered reassurance—holding her hand, letting her know that she now has the inner resources to cope with this memory—she might have been able to negotiate it more easily. This highlights the profound impact that psychedelic therapists' language and directives can have on trauma survivors.

SYMPATHETIC AND PARASYMPATHETIC RESPONSES

Our sympathetic nervous system initiates the "fight-or-flight" response, preparing the body for a rapid response to potential threats and danger. Another system is activated in this aroused state: the hypothalamic–pituitary–adrenal (HPA) axis. The release of stress hormones from the adrenals accomplishes many of the same effects as the sympathetic system: increasing heart rate, dilating airways, and directing blood flow to the skeletal muscles, all of which facilitate motor actions, such as running, pushing, and striking. These swift physiological changes are crucial for survival, enabling immediate, decisive action and enhanced physical performance in stressful situations.

Once the threat has passed, the parasympathetic nervous system helps restore calm with its characteristic "rest and digest" response. The neurotransmitter acetylcholine facilitates recovery by downregulating autonomic functions, such as heart rate, respiration, and muscle tension. The sympathetic and parasympathetic systems are designed to function in opposition to each other.

SOCIAL ENGAGEMENT SYSTEM

The parasympathetic system also supports social engagement behaviors (Porges, 2011). This promotes cooperation among mammals, fostering deeper social bonds. Activation of the social engagement system triggers the release of oxytocin and vasopressin—which enhance feelings of trust and connection—and helps mitigate stress responses by promoting relaxation and a sense of ease. This improves individual well-being and enhances group cohesion and survival as cooperative social structures are better equipped to face environmental challenges.

A central role of the ANS is maintaining homeostasis by regulating bodily functions, keeping them within an optimal range for different environmental conditions. When trauma occurs, the ANS's ability to maintain homeostasis can become disrupted. If environmental stressors are chronic or severe, the ANS may struggle to return to its baseline state, leading to habituated states of hyperarousal or collapse. In other words, the fight, flight, or freeze response doesn't turn off once the threat has passed—the alarm system stays on, the body primed for danger.

TRAUMA AND MEANING MAKING

These nervous system states shape our cognitive and emotional responses. Driven to make meaning in our lives, the narratives of trauma survivors can severely limit their prospects. Early trauma can be profoundly damaging. Tronick's (2007) still-face experiment—which investigated infants' distress when exposed to unresponsive caregivers—highlights the critical role of emotional reciprocity in early development. Disruptions in caregiver interactions can significantly affect an infant's emotional regulation and attachment patterns.

When a parent is chronically depressed, their mood may imprint on the child's developing brain, influencing physiological functions. Intrusive or neglectful caregiver behavior can create stress and overwhelm for the developing child, establishing a disordered baseline for their psychophysiological state. Conversely, an emotionally attuned parent fosters a sense of well-being and trust, teaching the child that close relationships are a reliable source of support. These early interactions become the blueprint for engaging with the world. We make meaning from interactions with our caregivers, forming the basis of our intuitive responses to other people throughout our lives.

In psychedelic therapy, such deep-seated patterns of meaning making can resurface. Long-forgotten memories and preverbal emotional states frequently show up in journeys. Unusual body sensations and dreamlike imagery symbolically express this hidden web of meaning, which can be explored later in the integration stage (see Chapters 12 and 13). Understanding the role of trauma in our early relational patterns can provide insight into the beliefs and assumptions that shape a person's life.

TRAUMA AND THE PREPARATION STAGE

In the preparation stage, it is essential to assess how best to support the client if trauma memories surface in their journey. This includes establishing clear agreements around touch if trauma should emerge. We collaborate with the client, identifying the forms of support that will be helpful in moments of discomfort, tension, and anxiety.

The therapist should be aware of any significant traumas in a person's background, and we should ask them if confronting these traumas aligns with their intentions. Practicing somatic techniques—such as breathing, simple movements or stretches, and grounding exercises—can be beneficial. Familiarizing a client with these practices ensures that they can access and apply them during the therapeutic journey. When trauma is approached in the preparation stage with compassion, and resources are offered to cope with it if trauma should arise, clients are much better equipped to navigate challenging moments in their journey and make meaningful progress toward healing.

Try This: Exhale—a Lot!

This practice can be useful when tension and anxiety arise in a journey:

1. The client lies down comfortably, feeling the ground beneath and the support it offers.
2. Instruct them to exhale deeply, making an audible huff, as one might do before a dramatic complaint. They can accentuate this by flapping their lips.
3. The client should focus on exhaling forcefully, letting their weight drop into the earth as they do so. They may notice sensations of melting or release as they exhale.
4. If they feel the urge to laugh and be playful during this exercise, that's even better. Laughter is a powerful tool for dissolving tension and enhancing relaxation.
5. The goal is to introduce exhaling as a tool to regulate and release tension and anxiety.

TRAUMA IN THE JOURNEY STAGE

There are two divergent schools of thought about handling trauma that arises in a journey. The first perspective recommends nonintervention—allowing the client to experience the full intensity of their process without any interference. This approach relies on the therapeutic container and the psychedelic agent to do the healing, not the therapist. The belief is that the client will see what they need to see, feel what they need to feel, and that enduring the emotional charge of trauma in a journey is an important part of the healing process.

The second perspective advocates for strategic interventions—the therapist provides support when trauma arises in the journey. This may involve offering healthy touch, or reassuring words, to help the client through difficult moments. Such interventions titrate the intensity of the experience, help avoid overwhelm, and support the client in finding inner resources, all of which make surrendering to the journey more manageable. The challenge lies in balancing the need for intervention with respecting the natural course of any therapeutic process.

From our perspective, the therapist should consider the validity of both kinds of responses, seeing each as appropriate for different situations. Strategic interventions *do* help clients navigate challenging moments, helping to avoid retraumatization in the journey. A client once described her work with an underground psychedelic therapist as "having to endure internal abuse without adequate support." The lack of guidance from her guide left her feeling exhausted and fearful, and in the aftermath exacerbated her night terrors and flashbacks. In the end, the journey had made her symptoms worse. Incorporating somatic resourcing techniques into her preparation sessions could have significantly alleviated her distress, deepening the healing potential of her journey. At the same time, some people may benefit from having space to be with the terror of aloneness, or a sense of helplessness or futility. To fully live through these experiences, without them being antidoted by the therapist, may facilitate the emergence of a more profound sense of mastery. The key is knowing when to intervene, which may not always be obvious. To err on the side of checking in, making oneself available to hold a light for a journeyer in darkness, is probably wise.

Repressed memories can also arise in psychedelic journeys. After trauma, the psyche appears capable of taking memories offline, making them inaccessible to conscious recall. Some journeyers could discover elements of their life story they'd forgotten, or that were previously unknown to them. This can be extremely disquieting. The focus at these points should be on stabilization and grounding the journeyer in their body, in the here and now. They may be ready to process this memory, or it may need to be acknowledged and saved for another time. Taking a break to connect to the environment through the senses can be useful here, as we don't want to rush into anything.

Though the repression of memories does occur, the therapist needn't go hunting for repressed memories—particularly during psychedelic experiences. As discussed, the expanded state of consciousness is a highly suggestible state, one in which the mind becomes more porous. Our autobiographical memory, already a slippery proposition, can become less organized and coherent. Just as repressed memories are real, so are *false memories*. Suggesting to the journeyer that there is likely some hidden trauma in their history—an event that would surely explain their distress—may just create one.

New information emerging in the journey can indicate new directions to work, but it's important to understand that these may be creatively rendered symbols of a person's pain rather than empirically true recollections. An openness to the recovery of memory, tempered with an awareness that memory can be extraordinarily imprecise, will serve us well as we accompany people embodying their life story in the psychedelic state.

Try This: Pendulating From Activation to Resource

In this preparation practice, introduce your client to the technique of alternating their focus between a resource in the body and a place of activation (see Chapter 4, the "Pendulation" section). The goal is to observe how consciously bringing awareness to a resource can influence and downregulate activation. Here is a short script you can use with your client:

1. "Identify a positive or supportive sensation in your body—a sense of calm in your heart, a steady, even breath in your belly, or the feeling of your feet grounded on the floor."

2. "Now, think of a mild source of stress—nothing too intense, nothing related to your core trauma. Notice how your body is responding. Pay attention to subtle shifts, such as tightness or changes in your breathing. Observe these with curiosity."
3. "Now, redirect your attention back to the positive or supportive sensation. Observe how your body responds to this change of focus."

Trauma-Informed Interventions

When supporting a client through a distressing phase of the journey, interventions should be designed to help them trust their experience. To provide comfort and grounding, you can encourage them to focus on their breath, feel the support of gravity, or engage in simple self-touch. You can offer concise statements to guide them toward inner resources identified in the preparation stage. Avoid lengthy explanations or dialogue during these moments, saving those for the integration sessions. Clients might turn away from a distressing experience—your compassionate presence and gentle guidance will help them navigate through it.

Here are some examples of *guiding statements* that can help manage distress:

"I am right here with you. You are not alone."
"Remember your resource and trust yourself."
"Feel the support of the ground and connect with your [specific resource]."
"You are OK. Take a breath, allow yourself to make a sound, and move your body a little."
"It's OK to experience this right now. See what else is here for you."

The quality of the therapist's presence is paramount. It is essential to approach challenging moments calmly and with confidence. The client's suffering and intensity of emotion are integral parts of the therapeutic work, not problems to be immediately resolved. An effective therapist is one who can set aside any agenda around comforting the client, instead offering support for the process itself.

Another effective intervention when clients feel stuck is to change the music. While music can powerfully enhance the journey, intense or emotionally charged tracks can overwhelm a sensitive system. It's important to be mindful of this impact and to choose songs thoughtfully.

Observing the client's reaction to touch can tell us much about their relative state of relaxation or tension. During a ketamine session with a severely anxious client who was sharing an experience of violation with me [Manuela], I held her hand and guided her to breathe. Her initial hand clutching was desperate, but with the connection and containment—as well as my calm guidance and reassurance—she was able to relax, allowing the trauma to be processed more effectively. In the integration session, she shared that this had been profoundly healing. She felt her own vitality again.

Beneath the Unspeakable

Trauma therapists often bear witness to profound suffering: feelings of worthlessness, physical pain, and interpersonal mistrust. People share their degradation, the indignities they have borne. Beyond the mere application of therapeutic tools, we must cultivate genuine compassion and an ability to relate to suffering. In the oft-silent domain of trauma, where shame and guilt may suppress expression and freedom, psychedelic therapists foster a mindset of compassion and openness. This allows us to witness these difficult moments more fearlessly.

Trauma frequently occurs in secret. Describing it to a therapist can be terrifying but may be crucial for healing to occur. Sexual and physical abuse, in particular, often leave survivors with internalized messages of guilt, shame, and self-blame. During psychedelic experiences, this may manifest as previously incomplete body movements—such as fighting or fleeing, expressing taboo verbalizations, or reaching out for support—allowing individuals to articulate suppressed needs.

Therapists can interpret these motor programs as the mind–body complex, informing us what's been missing and what needs attention to heal.

Try This: Navigating the Challenge

Reflect on a client you've worked with who was particularly challenging. Recall the strong emotional charge you experienced in session with this client and the troubling stories you heard. As you bring this client to mind, pay attention to your immediate physiological response:

1. Observe whether there is any physical constriction or bracing in your body. Do you want to distance yourself from this client, or the emotions they evoke in you? Do you respond to this memory of them with compassion, or perhaps a sense of helplessness or ineffectiveness? Notice all of these initial reactions.
2. Now, imagine yourself releasing your reactions, allowing them all to sink down into the earth. Remind yourself that your role is to be present, not to fix or change anything.

3. Focus on adopting a quality of presence, without any need to "do" or intervene. Observe how your body responds to this attitude. What do you notice now?
4. You can jot down your observations in a journal entry and revisit this reflection whenever you have a strong emotional or physiological reaction to a client.

TRAUMA AND THE INTEGRATION STAGE

The 2-week period following a psychedelic experience is when the brain can most readily assimilate new information and form new habits (Nardou et al., 2019). For approximately 72 hours post-journey, subjects exhibit increased neurogenesis: the formation of new neurons (de Vos et al., 2021). Formal mindfulness practices can help stabilize these new connections, especially in the prefrontal cortex, which regulates impulse control and calms the amygdala's response to perceived threats (Davidson et al., 2003; Hölzel et al., 2011).

As mentioned, introducing somatic therapy techniques can be challenging for clients with significant trauma histories. In the immediate aftermath of a psychedelic journey, however, clients often become *more* receptive to body awareness. If this newfound openness to sensate experience is stabilized during integration sessions, it may prove to be enduring.

Additionally, clients should be encouraged to explore any inner resources that may have shown up in the journey. If a particular breath or movement practice helped them through a challenging moment, they may want to keep exploring this practice in daily life. One of my clients discovered a slow sequence of synchronized breathing and hand movements during her journey, reminiscent of a Balinese dance. Inspired by a mental image of a powerful female protector, this spontaneously emerging somatic resource helped her overcome a long-standing aversion to yoga. Eventually, she was led to a fulfilling career change in mental health.

The integration process helps clients recontextualize their trauma histories, allowing new perspectives from the journey to be brought into everyday life (see Chapters 12 and 13).

CONCLUSION

Trauma profoundly affects every aspect of subjective experience, influencing mental and physical health, relationships, and self-perception. While pain and suffering are inherent in the human experience, trauma does not have to be.

As clients navigate their unique paths toward relief and hope, they frequently encounter feelings of panic, isolation, helplessness, and hopelessness. The integrated use of psychedelic and somatic therapies offers a promising avenue for trauma recovery. By simultaneously addressing the mind, body, and spirit in the healing process, these approaches empower individuals to transform in lasting ways and reclaim their lives.

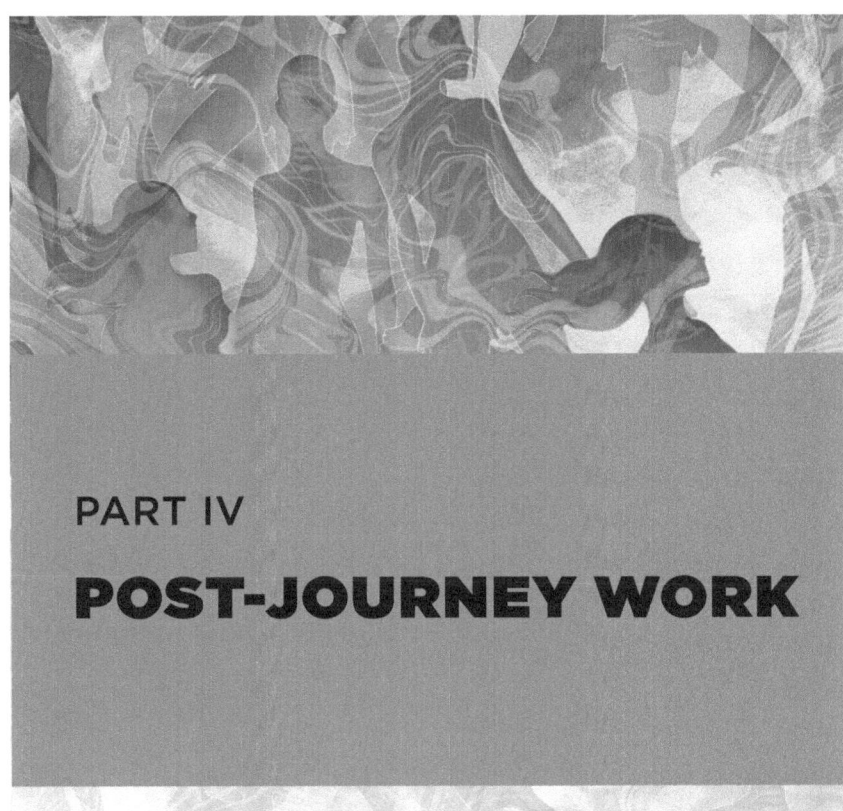

PART IV
POST-JOURNEY WORK

CHAPTER 12

What Is Integration?

*We do not choose a path. We can only take
the one that forms at our feet.*
—KEN MCLEOD

The process of "integration" after a medicine journey has become a cornerstone of psychedelic-assisted therapy. Integration is said to determine the therapeutic value of a psychedelic experience, but the term itself is often poorly defined. Let's demystify this process and explore how important the integration phase really is.

TRAUMA HEALING AS INTEGRATION

I [Joshua] discuss integration regularly in the trauma therapy trainings I lead. In recent years, the SE method has shifted from a *discharge model*—focused on the release of "trauma energy" trapped in the body—to an *integration model*—where overwhelming experiences can be renegotiated. In renegotiation, we allow the psyche to process through what is still incomplete from these past events, assimilating it into the totality of our being.

Neurobiological theories about trauma support this approach. While the neurological basis of PTSD is still being investigated, some researchers have drawn attention to *dissociated sensory frag-*

ments after intensely stressful events (Kearney et al., 2023). This describes the way particular elements of experience—say, the sound of screeching brakes, the smell of the battlefield, or the sight of a person's face contorted in rage—get lodged in our brains and are repeatedly played back, taking us out of the here and now and into the "there and then" of past trauma.

We have several distinct memory systems operating in our brain (Parkin et al., 1990). *Procedural memory* relates to learning that is *implicit*—not consciously recognized. Once we learn to ride a bike, we never forget. Our bodies somehow know how to do this complex thing, without conscious thought. This is an example of implicit memory.

Then there is *autobiographical memory*, or *explicit* memories that we record throughout our lives. Autobiographical memory, sometimes called *narrative memory*, is our recollection of what has occurred in the past, accessible to conscious retrieval.

In trauma, overwhelming experiences create imprints in the procedural memory system, which are not consolidated into our narrative memory (Levine, 2015). These dissociated sensory fragments are stored in procedural memory circuits, randomly intruding into our awareness as highly charged somatosensory states. Because they never get processed and filed into our memory archive, they never recede into the past. They continue to overstimulate our nervous system, making us feel as if the past event is happening again, right now.

Much of trauma healing, then, involves integrating experiences that fragmented us. By carefully combing through these dissociated percepts, we confront unfinished aspects of experience—our soma processes the emotions, sensations, and movements it was unable to complete at the time, giving the nervous system the signal that the trauma is over: It's done, and we made it. We can go back to our lives with this event now in the past, still part of us, but only in memory. Trauma healing is a process of integration.

What does this mean for psychedelic work? As we've seen, the psychedelic experience has value to the extent that it transforms us. Expanded states reveal information about the deep self, our connection to the world and, potentially, worlds beyond. However, this torrent of intelligence will not change us unless it is sifted through, processed, and brought into daily life.

DISINTEGRATION IN THE MODERN WEST

Interestingly, integration practices aren't prominent features of the Indigenous medicine traditions (Aixalà, 2022). It may be that some cultures inherently facilitate more integrated ways of being. As mentioned, the discontinuity between altered states and daily life may be less pronounced in these societies, and so an explicit integration process is less necessary.

Modern Western cultures, on the other hand, tend toward fragmentation. In industrial civilization, the individual is atomized, separate. The epidemic of loneliness that plagues industrialized societies is a grim consequence of this globalized alienation. The chasm between ourselves and our fellows yawns ever wider as we increasingly live our lives online, the digital facsimile of life claiming more and more of our attention. Loneliness is known to damage health, shorten life expectancy, and create psychopathology (Putnam, 2020).

Some of us also experience *othering*: a distorted lens we are seen through, based on bias and stereotypes, causing us to be perceived as less than or "not normal." Our culture is increasingly stratified and hierarchical, with income inequality widening and various systemic inequities remaining pronounced. In this desolate social landscape, a sense of belonging can be hard to find.

We have also become largely disconnected from spirituality, with levels of religious participation dropping to record lows (Jones, 2021). Connection to nature is also imperiled, as wild spaces continue to be threatened by "development," becoming more and more difficult to access. The human organism evolved in communion with the wild—as Shepard (1982) wrote, "We suffer for want of that vanished world" (p. 15).

On top of this, we are alienated from our bodies. Inheritors of Cartesian dualism, we distrust our direct somatic life. We tend to value abstract cognition over emotion and sensation, seeing the body as a *thing* controlled by the mind. We equate safety with control, and financial success is often predicated on our willingness to override impulses and domesticate our longings.

Our world is becoming speedier and more intense all the time. We rush through our day frenetically, pushed from one task to the next without pause. This rhythm, out of keeping with our evolutionary continuum, prevents us from integrating experience. Without time to stop and reflect, we carry a backlog of unprocessed experiences that dwell in the unconscious, giving rise to anxiety, depression, and a chronic dissociation from the present moment.

WHAT IS INTEGRATION?

So, we've established that integration is important, particularly in the modern West, but what *is* integration? The word itself carries different definitional meanings. Integration means taking something in, or incorporating a piece of something into a larger whole. We do this when we learn new things, assimilating novel information into our existing mental models.

Integration also means creating a new whole out of disparate parts. In a disordered psyche, divided against itself, mental processing has a chaotic quality, a lack of cohesion between differing motives and habits. As we saw in earlier sections on the *shadow*, the parts of ourselves that elicit shame often remain unintegrated. We are unaware—or mostly unaware—of these tendencies, until they erupt into unseemly behaviors.

To be integrated, then, is to be whole, to have assimilated a lifetime of experience into a coherent sense of self. Aware of our tendencies toward selfishness, it means that we hew closer and closer to our internal knowing of who we really are, what Winnicott (1965) called the *true self*. This allows for spontaneous authenticity, a state in which there is more congruence between our internal experience and external behavior. To be integrated is to be aware of the various crisscrossing currents of our inner life, channeling this awareness into a way of being that expresses our deepest values and aspirations.

Being integrated also means that we're in touch with our bodies. We can examine here a synonym for integration: "incorporation." Combining the Latin roots *in* ("into") and *corpus* ("body"), this word suggests that to incorporate is *to embody*. When we go into the body, and feel what's happening within our flesh, we gain a deeper knowing of who we are.

In fact, the integration of experience often changes our physiology. After an SE or Hakomi session, a person's posture may change. They may notice that a part of the body that had been chronically tense is now relaxed. The heartbeat may be softer, or slower, and the breath may be deeper and fuller. When we take things in, fully internalizing the moments in our lives, the body itself may take on a different shape. Integration is a process of becoming.

When we integrate, we clean the slate. We change our minds, and ready ourselves for the future. This is part of what happens during dreaming, when the unconscious sifts through our accumulated experience. In dreams, we live through experiences—or symbolized versions of them—with much of the emotional content siphoned off, as emotion processing centers of the brain are dampened during sleep (Goldstein & Walker, 2014). This allows the mind to make sense of and integrate experiences into our existing matrix of understanding. It is worth noting that trauma breaks down this process—sleep disturbance and recurrent nightmares are common posttraumatic symptoms (Koffel et al., 2016).

THE THERAPEUTIC VALUE OF INTEGRATION

When experiences are difficult to integrate, we must work to process the new information and weave it into ourselves. This is one of the hallmarks of effective trauma therapy, such as the Somatic Experiencing method. Because trauma is experienced in a nonordinary state of consciousness, trauma therapists reawaken elements of that prior state in order to make sense of the experience. We evoke *state-dependent memory*: by kindling the memory of a person's trauma we reestablish the mental state the person was in at the time, which unlocks embodied recollection of those moments (Rothschild, 2000). The original traumatic event then becomes more available for integration.

Psychedelic experiences are similar in that the relevant mental state is entirely unlike normal, waking consciousness. To make use of this extraordinary phenomenology, we must cultivate and safeguard a space for reflection, unpacking and absorbing the various revelations of the journey. This is the purpose of the integration session, conducted after the dosing session. In integration sessions we bring the lessons of the journey into the here and now, allowing us to change behaviors in our day-to-day life.

It is the psychedelic therapist's responsibility to open the door to the numinous *and* to *close* it. It's not enough to prepare a journeyer and hold space for their process; we must also facilitate its completion. Unlocking the realms of the human unconscious can be a great gift but we also need to welcome the journeyer back to the solid ground of ordinary life.

As we do this, the journey becomes something that occurred in the past. The client may continue to gestate and explore it, but the altered state itself has come to an end. Reestablishing stability and the reconstellation of one's normal experience is key. The journeyer may feel *different* but should not feel like a stranger to themselves.

Part of integration sessions will be recalling the journey, highlighting any significant shifts and insights that occurred. We celebrate the courage and fortitude that carried the client through their inner adventure. We also filter the experience for the client, recognizing what's important to focus on and what might have been extraneous noise from the conditioned mind (or "ego"). Journeyers are often relieved to have someone to help remember what happened and make sense of it, particularly if the content was surprising, confusing, or mysterious.

We can review the client's intention, investigating how it may or may not have figured into the work. Journeyers often delight in seeing the connection between their intention and the insights that unfolded. At other times, they may feel a sense of wonder that the intention seemed to have been waylaid completely, forgotten as the psyche pursued more pressing matters.

The therapist can share notes, combing through the many hours of the journey and reminding the client of what was said and done. Having a written record of this "time outside of time" is a major benefit of guided journeys. It's common for the therapist to read from their notes and hear the journeyer exclaim delightedly, "Oh right, I forgot all about that part!"

Additionally, the therapist can share their experience of the process. It can be gratifying for journeyers to hear how they may have affected their guide. As long as it doesn't distract from the work, the therapist's sober experience of the journey can be a bright star in the client's constellation of meaning. Learning the specific way the therapist was touched and moved by their process can deepen their trust in what happened.

EMBODYING INSIGHTS AND EXPERIENCES

The integration stage is where the rubber of psychedelic work meets the road. The therapist helps the client ascertain how the various insights and epiphanies of the journey can be actualized, facilitating shifts in behavior. Is there a new practice the journeyer could commit to?

Perhaps their renewed awareness of the interconnectedness of all life would be strengthened by time spent daily in nature. A new sense of connection with an ancestor, deity, or other transpersonal resource could be maintained through prayer or meditation, or a new altar could be created in their home to honor this relationship. Changing exercise routines or eating patterns could be part of honoring a newfound sense of embodiment.

Ultimately, the journey should be understood as an initiation into a deeper level of one's own inner knowing. However valuable this may be, it is only useful if it's actionable in some way. Thoughts, feelings, and sensory states will be experienced differently for a time after the journey—but old patterns will reassert themselves in due course. It is only through sustained conscious effort that one's life can shift in deeper, more sustainable ways.

It's important to note that all of this focus on shifting things, this dogged pursuit of transformation, might cause us to miss a critical aspect of the work: *Therapy is as much about acceptance as it is about change.* Though it may seem paradoxical, self-acceptance is the heart of personal growth. What we now consider *symptoms* were once our psyche's best effort to protect us, valiant attempts to stay whole and safe in a world that felt inhospitable. When we accept ourselves, we acknowledge that the thoughts and behaviors we judge—and might desperately want to be free of—once *made sense*, and initially arose as seemingly necessary strategies to protect ourselves from danger. We can accept that we've done the best we could do with the resources we had, as we tentatively open ourselves to trying out new ways of being in the world.

Clients emerging from a journey often recognize that another way of being is possible, and some generate long lists of things they need to change right away. However, this voracious hunger for change must be tempered with self-acceptance. Each of us is on a lifelong path of growth and discovery, and it isn't reasonable to expect ourselves to suddenly attain enlightenment, no matter how impactful a recent journey may have been.

It sometimes takes years to integrate a single psychedelic experience. Many people report that they are still processing material uncovered in journeys undertaken long ago. Our ordinary mental state tends toward constriction and control, focused on the necessities of daily existence and the small-minded goals of the ego. It is a formidable challenge to actually become the person a journey suggests we could be, and it may take us a lifetime to get there.

In fact, some researchers suggest that integration must be incremental if we want it to be sustainable, particularly if the journey is profound (Bathje et al., 2022). Slow, steady change is easier to sustain than sudden radical shifts. It can feel stifling to slowly chip away at maladaptive patterns, making measured behavioral changes over the course of months or years, but this is a surefire path to unlocking our full potential.

Also, the bigger an experience is, the more time it will take to integrate. It takes diligent work over an extended period to put such momentous insights into practice and remake our habitual patterns. The therapist should expect that more provocative experiences will require more integration sessions. Another dosing session is rarely advisable before the preceding one has been processed, and the client has settled into new modes of perception and action.

CHALLENGES WITH INTEGRATION

Sometimes integration gets complicated. The task may appear simple enough: Support the journeyer as they sift through and make use of their experience. However, clients may struggle to understand what occurred, or have complex emotional reactions postsession. A lifelong atheist may suddenly encounter a divine intelligence. A devout monotheist may contact a deity from outside their faith tradition. Our most cherished beliefs can be torn asunder by a single journey! Even if this is ultimately positive, it can feel bewildering and be destabilizing.

A phrase coined for this kind of experience is *ontological shock* (Argyri et al., 2024). Ontology is the study of being, encompassing our notions of existence and assumptions about reality. We order our lives with basic suppositions about what things mean, and what behaviors should result from these meanings. A psychedelic experience can turn this all on its head, giving us experiential proofs that things are not as they seemed. Though this may open pathways to new directions in life, it can still leave us floored and make daily life more difficult.

Medically speaking, shock is a response to perceived threat, involving shifts in bodily function and a concomitant alteration of one's psychological state. As our nervous system changes its pattern of response, we may feel disoriented and discombobulated.

Many journeyers find it difficult to "make room" for the enormity of a new truth, struggling to reconfigure their understanding of the world and their place in it. In other words, they may feel unsure of how to be a person who knows this new thing. The therapist can normalize the bewildering experience, reminding them that big changes take time to adapt to. As they say in 12-step programs, "Easy Does It."

The client may feel shame. This could be either a response to the content of the journey, or a sense of being unworthy of its sacredness. Psychedelics create vulnerability. In the altered state, people often say and do things that later—from the perspective of normal consciousness—seem regrettable or absurd. A client will be absorbed in the beauty and profundity of their journey, only to arrive at their integration session withdrawn and embarrassed the very next day. Clients may need the therapist to normalize any odd-seeming aspects of their experience, or even celebrate them. I [Joshua] tend to remind such clients that in this work we are given opportunities to meet new parts of ourselves, deepening our self-understanding and encountering the shadow. Shadow work is difficult, particularly encountering the shame associated with it, but this is one of the ways we put love into action: coming to know ourselves, warts and all, so we can accept and appreciate the unique being that we are. This allows us to see *other* people wholly, and reduces the likelihood that we'll act in harmful ways.

Another potential challenge to the integration process is the reaction of those around us. Our friends, family, or community may cringe at the earnestness and wonder on full display after a journey. They may denigrate the childlike openness many people feel after psychedelic therapy, or cast aspersions on the journey itself through judgment, dismissal, or doubt. It's hard enough for clients to endure their own self-doubt, trusting and honoring their psychedelic experience—let alone the skepticism of others! As mentioned in the "Preparation" section (see Chapter 7), it's crucial that journeyers know who they can talk with about their journey . . . and, perhaps, who they shouldn't.

Having a supportive community is crucial for integrating any major life event. The more we are surrounded by caring, compassionate people—who understand us and champion our growth and change—the better off we'll be. People emerging from psychedelic journeys are like newborn babies: dazed, tentative, open, and exquisitely sensitive. Clients will ideally have people around who are gentle and sincere, who can help the journeyer regulate, stabilize, and integrate. Would you trust this person with a baby? If not, maybe don't reach out to them!

Another post-journey complication is clients exhibiting what's called *ego inflation*: becoming convinced they are now somehow special, an emissary of an elect group, chosen to represent transpersonal beings or convey precious truths. They may evangelize, setting themselves above and apart from others, certain they've been charged with the task of saving those around them. This behavior is sometimes a transitory phase of overexcitement about the psychedelic-assisted change process, and will abate on its own. At other times, it continues long enough to *seriously* get on people's nerves. It smacks of spiritual materialism, as if one's personality has been supplanted by a new and improved "spiritual" façade. This can be understood as a kind of coping mechanism that requires time and work to dismantle, as painful, repressed emotions get processed.

LOOKING TO THE FUTURE

Therapists should caution their clients against making major life changes in the immediate aftermath of a journey. Clients often become convinced—in the course of their dosing session or after—that they need to quit their job, end their marriage, or in other ways radically transform their lives. Psychedelics can help identify the need to make changes, but it's rarely advisable for people to respond by upturning their life circumstances. In fact, the main objective of the first integration session after a journey is for the client to restabilize. Therapists can remind clients that life circumstances can always be reevaluated after the integration process is complete. Instead of inventing a whole new life, we can help them weave new insights into the life they already have. Pumping the brakes on radical change can feel somewhat counterintuitive, but it's a surer way to consolidate the therapeutic gains psychedelics afford.

As therapists, we may need to coordinate care with other helpers. If it doesn't violate a confidentiality agreement, the client can give consent for the psychedelic therapist to discuss the journey with a counselor, bodyworker, clergy person, or medical provider. It is always a wise policy to have trusted practitioners in our locale to whom we can refer clients for ongoing care.

Once we're confident the dosing session has been integrated and stabilization has occurred, the client may want to consider another journey. Remember, many of the landmark studies on psychedelic-assisted therapy involved multiple administration sessions (e.g., Davis et al., 2020; Mithoefer et al., 2011). It seems to be the case that repeated psychedelic experiences increase neuroplasticity, exponentially magnifying the therapeutic potential of these drugs. This is especially true if past journeys have been integrated thoroughly, readying the person to build upon the new foundation they've laid.

Appropriate spacing is critical here. While some research protocols with psilocybin involve consecutive dosing sessions a mere 2 weeks apart, many experienced underground guides suggest a minimum 3-month interval between journeys. In some cases, an even longer period may be necessary to integrate a particularly impactful dosing session. This needs to be handled with care, on a case-by-case basis, ensuring that each client is supported to make the correct choice for their unique situation.

CONCLUSION

Integration can be an elusive concept. It involves the assimilation of one's life experience into memory and sense of self, which facilitates personal change and growth. We are integrated, then, when we feel whole and awake, embodied and present in the here and now, not weighed down by accumulated experience we have not yet reckoned with.

In integration sessions, therapist and client sift through the content of a journey. We can apply body-centered approaches, drawing the client's attention to somatosensory cues that arise as they describe the journey. We can remind them that the insights they gained are likely to fade if not accompanied by shifts in daily habits. We emphasize that this can take time, and it's vital to not rush the process. Integration must be allowed to unfold organically, taking all the time it needs.

The therapist should caution the client not to change too much, or change too fast, even if they feel compelled to radically remodel their lives. Altering one's circumstances is best saved for after the integration stage. Once the journey has been fully processed, a deeper integration may involve another experience of the medicine. We want to be careful with the time interval, not exposing the person too soon to another potentially destabilizing experience (but also not waiting so long that any synergistic effects between journeys are lost).

As psychedelics continue to be demystified and become more fully integrated into the culture around us, it may be that we need less intensive practices following a journey. I'll leave you with a quote from Marc Aixalà (2017), who literally wrote the book on psychedelic integration: "The future of integration is that we no longer have to talk about it because the work is done; the future of integration is that we do not need integration" (para. 33).

CHAPTER 13

Therapeutic Tools for Integration

> *Not enough people feel that our consciousness, our minds, souls, ideals are intertwined with the earth in which we are embedded. As we become more aware of this intertwining, perhaps there is some hope that we will succeed in turning away from destruction.*
> —DON HANLON JOHNSON

The integration phase is crucial for clients committed to change. This process can span weeks, years, or even decades. In fact, my [Manuela] client once processed an overwhelming psilocybin experience from her teenage years—20 years later. Her inquiry into this trip allowed her to make new meanings about the past, unpacking a compartmentalized event and making use of it. Through integration work, she reconnected with her younger self, a young woman in her late teens, buckling under the weight of new responsibilities: becoming a single mother, entering the workforce, struggling with addiction, and putting her baby up for adoption. The childhood trauma that surfaced in her teenage mushroom trip had been too much for her to handle. She had made many bad choices avoiding that pain. However, the decades-old imagery returned in one of our somatic therapy sessions, facilitating the integration of her experiences. This allowed her to release the shame and self-blame she'd been carrying all those years.

Many clients seek out psychedelics in order to transcend suffering. They often say something like "I want to change; I don't like my life." They expect psychedelics will increase their sense of well-being, making life easier to bear.

What they don't quite seem to realize is that the change process is *hard*. It requires a commitment to facing the shadow, letting go of attachments, and forgiving ourselves and others—even when things seem unforgivable. Without a willingness to face adversity, we risk falling into *spiritual bypassing*. This term was introduced by psychologist and meditation teacher John Welwood (2000), describing how some people use spirituality to avoid the messiness of life, antidoting their pain by escaping into spiritual ideals. They talk themselves out of suffering by explaining everything away as an illusion—or meditate in an effort to disappear into a sanctified realm of dissociation, rather than using mindfulness as a way to embrace their lived experience. Those engaged in spiritual bypassing are sometimes drawn to psychedelics, seeing them as a ticket out of accepting their earthly existence, their frailties and failings.

Integration is serious work, best approached in manageable steps—one insight, one practice, one deciphered image at a time. After a journey, clients have increased access to their inner life for a time. The new thoughts, feelings, sensations, and symbols can now inform their decisions, making them more curious—as well as more accepting of life's challenges.

This chapter provides practical tools for therapists who support people through the integration phase. Each client digests and assimilates experience uniquely. Below, we detail some practices applicable to a wide variety of situations.

PHASES OF INTEGRATION

Following a journey, the brain is primed for metamorphosis. Neuroplasticity is increased, with synaptic growth and increased connectivity fostering the development of new neurobiological pathways (de Vos et al., 2021). The most notable behavioral shifts usually occur in the days and weeks after a journey. But, as mentioned, integration can continue for months—or even years.

We propose approaching integration in three phases: an initial stabilization phase; a phase of focused work; and a longer-term, future-oriented phase.

> *Phase 1*: Immediately after the journey, the therapist encourages the client to let things settle. We coach them to document their experience while it's fresh, capturing all the phenomena and insights without any pressure to make sense of it. Maintaining an attitude of openness is essential, as deeper meanings will unfold over time. Suggest that your client practice mindfulness, gentle embodiment practices, and time in nature, letting the mind and body come back to Earth.
>
> *Phase 2*: In the phase of focused work, support your client to actively work with any insights through focused embodiment practices, dream work, journaling, psychotherapy, meaningful conversations, meditation practice, movement, making art, and introspection. Engaging with the content of the journey allows new meanings to take shape.
>
> *Phase 3*: To conclude the formal integration process, discuss with your client how to commit to lasting change. Establishing new habits—such as diet or lifestyle change, a daily mindfulness practice, or a new hobby—

scaffolds the creation of a new identity structure, a new way of being.

After these integration sessions, the process can continue indefinitely, assisted by the therapist or other supportive individuals. It can also arise out of self-directed inquiry. Some insights from a journey may become clear only after daily habits are modified. The ultimate goal is for the lessons of the psychedelic experience to facilitate a sustainable shift of being.

Of course, if you only plan on having one integration session—or two—these phases may unfold with some simultaneity. Let journeyers know that they shouldn't pressure themselves afterward. At some point, though, they should begin actively engaging with the material. This will naturally lead into a process of inquiry, translating these new perspectives into commitments, transforming their daily living in ways that honor the gifts they've been given.

IMMEDIATELY AFTER A JOURNEY

In the days after a journey, clients need to nourish their bodies. Eating cleanly, prioritizing sleep, and spending time in nature will be supportive. Unfocused activities can allow for continued processing. You can encourage the client to try automatic drawing—putting pen to paper and seeing what comes out—even if they don't consider themselves artists. Freewriting, the unstructured spilling of words onto a page with no editing or organization, can also be revealing. They need to create conduits for the unconscious to continue expressing itself, consolidating what emerged in the psychedelic state.

For the first few days after a journey, it's best to rest, be attentive, and simplify life. You can remind clients that they have the right to keep their process private, even from close friends or partners. It can be important to cherish the sacredness of the journey before attempting to share it.

FOCUSED WORK

As this initial period of recuperation gives way to the next phase, we invite clients to start actively exploring the material from the journey. Some of the following tools may prove useful.

Journaling

Therapists should encourage clients to write down everything they can recall from the journey. It's best if this happens the very next day. People are often amazed by how quickly the experience starts to fade, and important details can be lost if not captured early on. We can also encourage clients to reflect on their process using prompts, like the following:

1. What was the theme of the journey? If it had a theme song, what would it be?
2. What highlights of the experience stand out right now?
3. What images emerged during the journey?
4. Which guides, allies, or spirits showed up, if any?
5. What messages did I receive, or what insights am I experiencing now?
6. What surprising new thoughts and feelings have arisen?
7. What moments made me laugh or cry?

Intentions

Therapists can ask clients to revisit their intentions, evaluating how these shaped—or didn't—what happened. As they actively reflect on the experience, the therapist can ask how the insights of the journey align with their original goals.

Remind clients to approach this with an open mind. The following is a reflection exercise you can use to guide them in revisiting their intentions:

Try This: Revisit Intentions

1. Take a moment to recall what you aimed to achieve with this journey. Notice if you struggle to remember, or if there are too many competing messages. Or, perhaps, if you feel like you crammed too many different intentions into your journey.
2. Now, reread the intentions you wrote down. Do they seem congruent with what unfolded in your session? Was anything revealed that aligns with these ideas? If not, are you feeling disappointed or misaligned with your intentions?
3. Allow your body to settle and find stillness. Ask yourself: Given what I now know, what does my intention reveal? What is the essence of my intention at this moment? Write down whatever arises.
4. Where do these new intentions lead you? *Exit intentions* facilitate a sense of continuity. What are you bringing forward into your life? It's fine for it to be abstract, there's no need for concreteness. Trust your intuitive insights.

Emotional Integration

Psychedelics release emotion, at times to an extreme degree. Identifying the emotional themes of the journey can generate valuable insights, helping journeyers deepen their self-awareness and enrich their inner life.

Research by Paul Ekman (2003) highlights the importance of accurately recognizing our emotions. This can enhance emotional intelligence, improve communication, foster deeper connections with others, and increase societal harmony.

Clients may be surprised at what gets evoked as they think about the journey. They may be despondent or hopeful, filled with gratitude toward the world or angry about how they've been treated in their lives. Accessing the physical sensation associated with a particular emotion can deepen the feeling while also containing the experience.

Try This: Befriending Difficult Emotions

In this practice, you're invited to explore an emotion you wish to understand better, whether it's anger, grief, shame, or anxiety.

1. Begin by choosing the emotion you want to delve into. Try to get a sense of it as an external entity, an energy with its own personality. Consider what this emotion would look like if it were a person.
2. Next, think about how this person behaves and interacts with the world. How do they move? Are they fast and erratic, or slow and heavy? What kind of voice do they have? Do they indulge in comfort food, throw things, or curl up with a book?
3. As you imagine this person sitting before you, notice your physical response. What sensations arise in your body? Do you feel tense, relaxed, or something else? Does this person remind you of a specific memory or situation? How do you feel about them?
4. Extend a hand toward this person (you can do this physically as well). Speak to them, saying, "I'm curious about

you . . . what would it take for us to be friends?" Observe their reaction. What do they say or do? Do they have any demands or conditions for friendship? What do they need from you?

5. Try to truly receive their response. What insights come up right now? How do things shift? What happens to you on an emotional level?

6. Take a moment to express gratitude to the entity you met. Did you notice this embodiment of the emotion change? How might this understanding help you in the future?

Embodied Movement

Coming more fully into the body will be a major asset in the integration phase. Mindfulness practice, breathwork, authentic movement, yoga, qigong, and countless other practices strengthen our body and sensitize our minds. Embodiment encourages authentic expression, allowing people to process experiences more holistically.

Try This: Following Impulse

1. Recall a moment from your journey that you wish to explore further. Try to remember the music that accompanied this moment, perhaps even replaying a particular song if you know it by name. Bring back the thoughts, images, and feelings, and then exhale sharply, releasing your body into the rhythm you feel.

2. If movement is new to you, start with a gentle swaying motion to get yourself going. Allow your body to move organically, following its natural impulses.

3. There's no script here; let go of any agenda and follow what feels right in the moment. Move with the image or archetype you encountered during your journey, allowing yourself to embody that part of yourself or to dance in partnership with it.
4. Explore and pay attention to the subtle impulses in your body. As feelings and sensations arise, allow yourself to continue moving, assimilating them as you go. Remember, life is in constant motion, and your body mirrors this.
5. Afterward, take some time to write and reflect on what came up. Pay attention to the quality of your awareness after the practice. How do things feel now?

Dreamwork

Anecdotally, we've seen many journeyers report a more vivid and detailed dream life—as well as better dream recall—after psychedelic experiences. Dreamwork homes in on the enigmatic symbols of the unconscious, some of which may have first emerged in the journey itself. We explore and interpret them in various ways to deepen the journey's insights. In the integration phase, dreams often explicitly connect with the content of the journey.

Jung (1934/1970) wrote, "The dream is a little hidden door in the innermost and most secret recesses of the soul" (p. 144). Paying more attention to messages from dreams and remembrances from our journey brings us into greater alignment with our deep self. In the modern world, symbols have largely lost their significance, being seen as simple signifiers rather than archetypal containers of meaning. We see an image in a similar way as we would a word on a page, an empty vessel linked to an abstraction. To more deeply penetrate into hidden content, take time to explore your emotional responses beyond words and associations. You can do this through journaling, drawing, movement, or simply sitting mindfully, exploring what comes through as you engage with symbolic forms. Allow unique meanings to be revealed as you meet these images on their own terms. Trusting the unconscious starts with an openness to dream images and listening to its mystery.

Try This: Dream Image

To work with your dream images, draw them or write about them, with no concern for representational accuracy. While digital imagery tools can be enjoyable, we recommend using traditional materials like paper, pens, pastels, and paints, creating an unmediated link to the mind and a rich sensorial experience as you interpret your dreams.

1. Sit quietly and recall an image from a dream—or a moment from the journey—you're curious about. Gather as many details as possible: colors, textures, size, shape, and adornments. No detail is too small. If you choose to draw, focus on capturing the essence of the image rather than a realistic or accurate representation. Prioritize free expression over precision.
2. If you prefer to write, approach the dream image as if it were a character. Let them speak in the first person, introducing themselves to you. Ask them:
    - "Who are you?"
    - "What brings you here?"
    - "What message do you have for me?"
    - "Is there something you want me to know?"

3. Write for 10–20 minutes without editing. Reread your work and notice what stands out to you. You can repeat this process with different elements of dreams or other moments from your journey.

Art

The field of art therapy has shown that drawing, painting, or sculpting can catalyze enduring change. A common practice in psychedelic integration is drawing mandalas—symbolic representations of inner and outer realities, often featuring concentric circular motifs. This geometry often captures psychedelic experiences with greater fidelity than words ever can. Even a coloring book can create openings into a sense of embodied ease and presence.

Simple crafts, such as cross-stitch or paint by number, can be quite relaxing, allowing space for inner experience. Craft has always been part of our human experience, as people engaged with the physical world through their hands. Weaving together strands of fabric, as one would in knitting or crochet, is a potent metaphor for the process of integration. Busying one's hands in a simple but engaging task frees up the mind to gestate experience, perfect for this phase.

Music

Singing, the archetypal human expression, opens a vibrational pathway to one's insides, allowing the body to embrace the world through the voice. Playing an instrument, or even drumming on a table, honors the body's urge to express itself. Spending some time strumming a guitar—or singing along with recorded music—might increase a sense of participation in the rhythms of embodied existence. Simple vocalizations, such as humming, reciting a mantra—or simply making any sounds that feel good—can be very helpful. The vibrations from these sounds positively impact our mood. All of these practices can be useful integration practices. We can encourage clients to make time for unstructured musical exploration, knowing this will be time well spent.

ONGOING SUPPORT FOR INTEGRATION

The final, future-oriented phase of integration comes next. At this point, the journey has been thoroughly combed through. Themes have been identified and explored in the body, mind, and soul. Now the journeyer continues to bring the experience into day-to-day life.

Invite the Client to Reflect

We begin by emphasizing that a full integration process takes time. Allowing space for reflection is essential. Remind the client that puzzling moments, conflicting feelings, or confusing images may require patience to understand fully.

Encourage Journaling

The therapist can suggest that clients continue the practice of reflective writing, perhaps keeping a journal dedicated to their journey and its aftermath. We encourage clients to regularly revisit their entries—especially the narrative of the journey itself—contemplating what they've written and how it might be incorporated into ongoing therapeutic work.

Reinforce New Habits

Therapists should discuss the importance of reinforcing new perspectives and beliefs by cultivating new habits. Invite clients to regularly remind themselves of their insights, perhaps placing notes around the house or listening to the music from their journey.

Create Meaningful Rituals

As clients navigate intense emotions or disorienting thoughts, suggest that they create rituals to symbolize the transitions they're undergoing. Invite them to pay attention to their food habits and media consumption, offering reminders that distractions pull us away from our authentic path. A daily ritual can increase their awareness of the transformation occurring within.

Engage Creativity

Encourage clients to enrich their creativity and explore new activities. Is there a new hobby they can take up, perhaps something they've been wanting to do but haven't made time for? We can offer the possibility that, over time, memories from their journey will resurface like sunken treasures, calling them back to their inner world again and again.

ABIDING IN STILLNESS

Creating time and space for stillness is essential in the integration phase. In stillness, we can hear the whispers at the edges of consciousness. Stepping away from the habitual drive to make sense of things invites us into greater expansion and openness. True integration requires us to rest in the present moment, opening to the underlying currents of change already tugging at us.

After a journey, the mind is more open. We can revel in this spaciousness, celebrating the new possibilities the space affords—or even feeling awe at the vastness of space itself. For effective integration, it's vital to be present with what is occurring in the here and now—rather than planning the next step. Abiding in stillness gives us the space to listen and be receptive.

Try This: Stillness in the Body

1. Find a comfortable position, either seated or lying down. Close your eyes and take a few deep breaths. Allow your breath to fall into a natural rhythm.
2. As you begin to settle, drop your attention into your body. Notice any areas of tension or discomfort. Imagine releasing that tension with each exhale, allowing your body to relax more deeply.
3. Visualize a warm, calming light enveloping you, starting at the top of your head and slowly moving down to your toes. Allow this light to soothe your muscles with each breath, bringing a sense of stillness.
4. As you breathe in, invite that stillness deeper into your being. With each exhale, release any distractions or worries. Feel the calm spreading through your body.
5. Stay in this stillness for a few moments, allowing yourself to just be.
6. Notice any sensations without judgment. If thoughts arise, acknowledge them and gently return your focus to your breath and the soothing light. Allow your mind to rest in this stillness, like a quiet winter day.

7. There is nothing to do, nothing to strive for—just be. Mark this feeling of stillness in your body, as if bookmarking it for future reference.
8. When you feel ready, gradually bring your awareness back to the room. Wiggle your fingers and toes, slowly opening your eyes. Take a moment to notice how your body feels now compared to when you began. Try to carry this stillness with you throughout your day, remembering you can return to this peaceful place whenever needed.

SHAME AND THE FURY OF THE PROTECTORS

Psychological "protectors" are one way of conceptualizing the aspects of self that help manage feelings of vulnerability, likely stemming from early-life experiences in which we felt unsupported. After deep, transformative work, feelings of shame and fear can resurface, leading to doubts and insecurities about what transpired in the journey. Clients may feel intensely exposed, grappling with what Brené Brown (2007) has called the *vulnerability hangover*.

Case Study: Sharon

After her first MDMA session, Sharon encountered deep-seated shame linked to her history of sexual trauma. Having felt disconnected from her body for years, she'd battled an eating disorder as a teenager, often hiding her slender frame in baggy clothes to avoid attention. She longed for freedom from the perceived limitations of her body. Any sensual feelings or body sensations would trigger uncomfortable memories of her trauma, which left her feeling exposed once she left the safety of the therapy room.

During her session, Sharon uncovered her anger at feeling stifled and overpowered, leading to a volcanic upwelling of rage and aliveness she had never experienced before. She began to dance with intense feeling, responding to the music with forceful movements. Afterward, tears of gratitude streamed down her face as she embraced her new sense of self. "I feel like a cat," she exclaimed, describing the joy of movement and sensation in her body.

However, during our first integration session, Sharon returned in her familiar baggy clothes, her emotional tone muted. As we debriefed, she expressed regret for her uninhibited movements, feeling embarrassed about how it must have appeared. Her *shame protectors* were activated, making her feel overexposed.

"It was a lot, huh?" I said.

"Yeah, I loved it, but I don't know what to do with it now. It feels overwhelming."

"Let's explore the parts of you that are present right now," I [Manuela] said. "It seems there's a feeling accompanying that overwhelm."

"I feel ashamed," she admitted, her lips pursing as if she'd swallowed something bitter.

"Let's make some room for that shame and see what it's saying," I offered.

"I can get in trouble if I'm that wild," she said, recognizing that her shame was trying to protect her. As we delved deeper, she identified a tightness in her lower belly.

"Is it okay to place your hand there and welcome the tightness along with the shame?"

She nodded, the disgust on her face more pronounced. "I'm really angry right now."

"That anger surfaced in your journey too. What kind of anger is it?"

"The kind that could be dangerous to others if I let it out."

I encouraged her to feel just some of that anger and notice what the tightness was doing.

"It's pushing," she said. "Wanting to push out and away."

I gave her space to allow that movement to happen.

After several strong exhales Sharon's eyes opened wide. "I'm so mad that my sensuality was taken from me, and shame was left to bear it all." She began pushing with her hands and legs, drawing on the sense of power she'd felt in her journey. She laughed. "In the journey I felt like I could push boulders around, like Wonder Woman."

"Let's connect with that feeling now so you can recognize it when shame returns."

She shook her head. "When I'm angry, the shame doesn't stand a chance. When I was little I couldn't express my anger. I would've been punished."

"Exactly. And how does the shame feel now?"

"Shame kept me small and hidden, like my Wonder Woman went into hiding."

I nodded. "Makes sense, given your history. How is that tightness in your belly now?"

"It's not there at all," she said. "I actually feel pretty strong."

"How can we support that strength?"

"I want to tell my little Wonder Woman that she doesn't need to feel ashamed anymore."

In our subsequent sessions, we continued to work on befriending anger, rage, and shame. Over time, Sharon's feelings of shame eased, and her attitude toward her body changed dramatically. She began to enjoy embodiment practices, and whenever feelings of shame arose, she recognized them as invitations to reconnect with her journey. She took up yoga, consciously moving and embracing her body in new ways.

Try This: Meeting the Protectors

These are some writing prompts you can use when shame comes up for your client. Remember that shame is an unprocessed emotion and a somatic state. While it is one of the most unpleasant emotions to feel, it is one that we need to connect with:

1. Begin by acknowledging the shame. Sit quietly and take a few mindful breaths, connecting with any sense of spaciousness in your body and mind. Then, ask yourself, "What is the opposite of shame?"
2. As you pose this question to yourself, remain open and avoid feeding into any story about the shame. Allow the answer to arise naturally. It may not come right away, but simply asking creates space for new insights to emerge. You may be completely surprised, or amused, by what your mind comes up with as shame's opposite.
3. Once you've given yourself time to reflect, grab your journal and write down your thoughts. Engage with the prompt for 10–20 minutes, letting your responses flow freely. This process can reveal new perspectives and cultivate gratitude.

GRATITUDE

The psychedelic journey is a personal experience, inextricably linked to how we perceive ourselves and engage with our lives. A frequent outcome of this work is the emergence of gratitude: for people, for the world, for our very existence.

Research shows that feelings of gratitude enhance mental and physical health, strengthen relationships, and foster emotional resilience (Wood et al., 2010). Practicing gratitude can improve sleep (Wood et al., 2009), as well as lower blood pressure and improve heart health (Cousin et al., 2020). Gratitude is a social glue, promoting prosocial behavior and building community bonds (Algoe, 2012).

The profundity of psychedelic journeys can usher in a cascade of beneficial effects, mediated by the experience of awe (Keltner, 2023; Monroy & Keltner, 2022). By initiating us into wonder, these powerful experiences can inspire gratitude and humility. The experience of awe reminds us that, in the grand scheme of things, our worries and doubts aren't that important.

Introduce your client to the practice of gratitude through journaling. The exercise below is a good way to start:

Try This: Gratitude Journal

Take some time to reflect on the moments of gratitude you experienced during your journey or in the following integration. How did this feeling resonate in your body?

Prompts:

1. What has the journey shown me, that I'm grateful for?
2. What am I grateful for in this moment?
3. Where do I get stuck when practicing gratitude?
4. How can I invite more gratitude into my life?
5. What small ritual of gratitude can I incorporate into my daily routine?

Allow your thoughts to flow freely as you write, and remember that this practice can deepen your connection to gratitude and enhance your overall well-being.

CONCLUSION

Clients are often eager to make good use of their journey, and will benefit from an attentive therapist's support in the integration phase. There is no one-size-fits-all approach to this process, and therapists need to trust their intuition, creatively facilitating integration for the particular client. Integration is itself a kind of journey—an unfolding, creative process that opens opportunities for embodiment, emotional depth, and greater cognitive coherence.

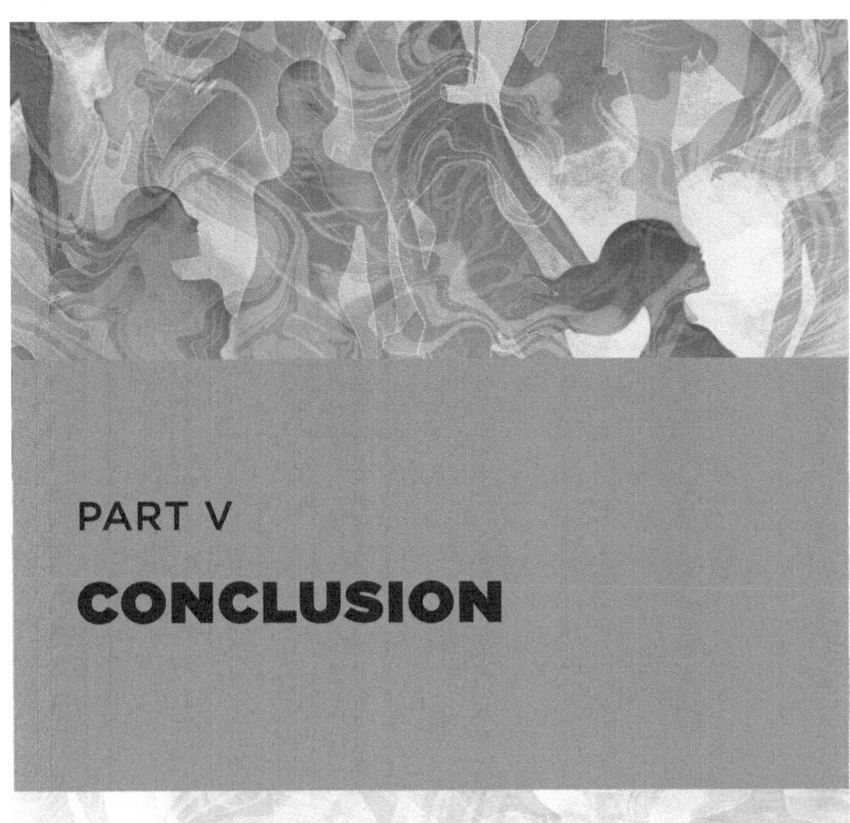

PART V
CONCLUSION

CHAPTER 14

Cultural Set and Setting

*There is a world beyond ours, a world that
is far away, nearby and invisible.*
—MARIA SABINA

THE PSYCHEDELIC POST-RENAISSANCE?

At the time of this writing, the "psychedelic renaissance" is in flux. With concern growing about the design of psychedelic studies, public health agencies are expressing mistrust. Clinical trials with thousands of subjects have established the efficacy of MDMA-AT in treating PTSD, for instance, yet MDMA is still classified as a Schedule I drug. The Drug Enforcement Administration (DEA) defines Schedule I as any substance that has "no currently accepted medical use and a high potential for abuse."

Yet, the medical usefulness of psychedelics seems obvious. Over 130 rigorously designed scientific studies on psilocybin alone have been published in the past two decades, and while the evidence remains clear that it can help depressed people at least as well as Lexapro can (Erritzoe et al., 2024), it still remains deadlocked in Schedule I. Clinicians eager to safely and legally utilize these medicines are left in the lurch.

The legalization of psychedelic therapy is important and necessary, both to make these treatments more widely available, and to create regulatory frameworks that protect consumers. In the current prohibitionist environment, unregulated guides operating in the black market can do a tremendous amount of damage, leaving clients no recourse to redress abuses.

Sexual boundary crossings continue to plague the public image of psychedelics. These violations have occurred at study sites, as well as in the underground. The most famous example, from a MAPS-sponsored study in Vancouver, Canada, involved a researcher initiating a sexual relationship with a study participant. This misconduct resulted in the journal *Psychopharmacology* retracting three prominent papers, all of which detailed robust evidence for MDMA in treating PTSD. *Psychopharmacology* never disputed the data. But because they were not informed of the transgression before the authors submitted their research, the journal took the extraordinary step of retracting publication—quite rare in academia. It is clear that sexual wrongdoing in psychedelic therapy is still a major concern.

Boundary crossings happen, and have always happened in therapy. We should be vigilant to this possibility, and do everything we can to safeguard the autonomy and dignity of clients. But the harsh reality is that no helping profession can be scrubbed clean of these stains. No less a figure than Carl Jung had an inappropriate sexual relationship with at least one patient (McLynn, 2014). State licensing boards overseeing mental health professionals receive scores of complaints each year, many of them related to sexual or romantic relationships between therapists and their clients.

Some claim that the pathology of exploiting people under the influence of psychedelics is uniquely Western. One need only review the many accounts of boundary violations from Amazonian ayahuasqueros, though, to see that such disfigured relationships to power transcend culture. Pseudo-shamans in the Global

South routinely abuse journeyers, leaving scars on their psyche, damaging their trust in others, and corrupting their relationship with these medicines.

By detailing the ubiquity of these abuses, we don't mean to normalize exploitation and harm, and we remain optimistic about making these ruptures less common. We want to foster a psychedelic culture that helps each person develop a bedrock of ethics, founded on a lasting commitment to protect the client in the complex relational dynamics of psychedelic therapy.

There are many guides in the underground who do practice in an ethical way. Indeed, their ethics are so strong that they risk their livelihood—even their very freedom—to make these treatments safely available. Other practitioners require oversight and accountability. Without someone looking over their shoulder, they may fall prey to their own avarice, lust, or egomania, making clients worse instead of better.

We understand why some people feel skeptical about government oversight of psychedelics. When it comes to therapeutic outcomes, however, having a structure for governance appears to be necessary. We no longer live in the small, tight-knit communities our ancestors enjoyed, in which everyone knew one another, and natural systems of accountability were in effect. In today's vast population of strangers, a board legislated to keep tabs on practitioners can protect clients and safeguard good outcomes.

There are unique ethical considerations concerning expanded states of consciousness. For instance, it is quite easy for psychedelic therapists to become grandiose. To a client on mind-altering drugs, the therapist may seem especially profound, even magical or divine. Many psychedelic therapists in the underground have become self-styled gurus, developing cultish followings. No longer accountable to anyone but their own loyal followers, they easily lose their moral compass. Some forget that they are simply stewards of the medicine, and come to see *themselves* as the healing force benefiting clients.

For all these reasons, and others, we look forward to a time when psychedelic therapy is legal and widely available. We hope that the burgeoning culture of psychedelic work develops a critical, self-reflective capacity, prioritizing the well-being, safety, and autonomy of those it serves. Continuing research will surely be helpful here, as we zero in on which factors create the best outcomes. A body-centered focus is one of these variables, and we hope this will be carefully researched in the years to come.

As the momentum of the psychedelic renaissance shifts, observers are left wondering where things will go next. Hopefully, this moment provides an opportunity to reflect, engage in dialogue and inquiry, and discover together what steps to take next.

THE REINTEGRATION OF INDIGENOUS WISDOM

In Western culture, there is a bias that each new innovation affirms the superiority of modernity. Congruent with this, we continue to see a widespread assumption that psychedelic therapies have been "discovered" by modern researchers. The same trend can be seen in the standard narrative of the founding of the United States—participatory democracy is solely credited to European influence, even though the U.S. Senate has admitted that many of the ideals and precepts that informed the Constitution originated with the Haudenosaunee, better known as the Iroquois Confederacy (H. Con. Res. 331, 1988).

Simply put, psychedelic healing practices are not new. They are by no means "novel treatments," nor any kind of "revolution." Humans have been altering consciousness in structured ceremonial frameworks for a long, long time. We have certainly done it for centuries, very likely for millennia, and possibly since before the time *homo sapiens* speciated. Some have even speculated that human consciousness itself—so clearly oriented toward religiosity and mysticism—was crystallized in the crucible of expanded states (McKenna, 1992).

Sadly, the West has yet to adopt an attitude of humility toward primary cultures, those that have successfully lived on this planet for thousands—or hundreds of thousands—of years. This arrogant mindset predominates in the sciences, an ethnocentric chauvinism that industrial societies reflect *progress*. Even as the modern world decimates its habitat—the very ecosystems it depends on for survival—it continues to define itself as more evolved, while traditional earth-based societies that have lived sustainably in place for millennia are labeled "underdeveloped."

What remains largely unrecognized regarding psychedelics is that we're using ancient solutions for modern problems. Western psychedelic therapy is, in many ways, reinventing the wheel—and perhaps doing a poor job of it, making a wheel that could easily fail to transport our culture to a healthier place.

THE THORNY HISTORY OF PSILOCYBIN

In recent years, research into psilocybin has far outpaced the study of its cousins: LSD, mescaline, and DMT (Garakani et al., 2023). As a result, some U.S. states have legalized psilocybin-assisted therapy, and there's reason to hope more people will be able to access these treatments in years to come. But Western culture has a troubled history with psilocybin. This serves as a sobering case study of modernity's incessant exploitation of Indigenous societies.

The figure of Maria Sabina looms large in discussions of psychedelic mushrooms. This legendary Mazatec *curandera* (healer) trained in her people's healing tradition with the native Oaxacan

Psilocybe mexicana, building a reputation in her community as a first-rate practitioner. In 1955, amateur mycologist Robert Gordon Wasson traveled to Mexico in search of a psychoactive fungus he'd heard was still used in native religious rites. He made a connection with Sabina, observed her healing work, and was greatly impressed by her skills. After several visits she agreed to initiate him (and his wife, Valentina Wasson) into the mysteries of the *velada*, the Mazatec mushroom ceremony (Estrada, 1981).

Wasson (1957) subsequently published an article about this experience in *Life* magazine. This article contained the first printed reference to "magic mushrooms," and its publication spawned a surge of interest in psilocybin (particularly in the counterculture). Droves of Western seekers descended on Sabina's hometown of Huautla de Jiménez to experience the magic for themselves.

Eventually, the impacts of psychedelic tourism in Huautla de Jiménez made Maria Sabina despondent. The flocks of visitors to her remote highland village cared little about the ritual use and cultural context of these sacraments. Their sudden influx overwhelmed the community, creating chaos and bringing Sabina into conflict with her neighbors, who burned her house down and briefly jailed her, seemingly in retribution for bringing such misfortune to her people.

In later years it came to light that Wasson had lied repeatedly to Sabina. He first sought her services in feigned desperation to find his missing son, though his son was fine. Pretending to be someone in need, Wasson preyed on Sabina's commitment to help others. He then assured her he would not disclose her name or the name of her village—a promise he promptly broke upon publication of the article in *Life*. The Wassons rose to prominence as the "discoverers" of magic mushrooms, won awards and accolades, and were paid handsomely for their articles, books, and speaking engagements. Huautla de Jiménez, however, remained impoverished and fell into social discord. Sabina died in poverty, estranged from her community, sickened with regret for introducing Wasson to the mushrooms.

Stories like this abound. The traditional indigenous knowledge keepers are forgotten, while the Westerners who popularize their plant medicine practices attain wealth and fame. Even today, American venture capitalists are raking in dividends as the field of psychedelics explodes. Yet the communities that originated these traditions, hiding and preserving them through centuries of persecution by European missionaries, receive nothing.

What would it look like if these cycles of extraction and exploitation were broken? How could the drivers of the psychedelic renaissance give something back to native communities and their homelands? And if this were to somehow happen, might indigenous voices rise to the forefront of the movement? We don't mean to be prescriptive here, or to promulgate a particular response to these complex issues. One thing is certain, though: As psychedelic therapy moves further into the spotlight, it casts an even longer shadow. Our hope is that the psychedelic renaissance is willing to do its own shadow work, redressing these long-standing problems. The movement itself may fall apart if it doesn't.

THE DIVINITY OF PSYCHEDELICS

All traditional systems of working with psychedelics have a religious or spiritual quality; it's worth recognizing that humans have rarely used these substances with a narrow focus on personal healing. In most indigenous knowledge systems, the medicines themselves are seen as intelligent and sentient, connecting people with deities, ancestors, or the spirits of plants and animals. This mystical quality may be inherent to psychedelics, whatever the cultural context of their use, and psychedelic therapists should be prepared to support transcendent experiences. Each practitioner needs to find their own way of doing this. We needn't fabricate or engineer spiritual experiences for our clients, but we need to welcome them when they arrive—and they will.

The discourse on psychedelics is too often medicalized, reduced to the treatment of psychopathology and the healing of personal trauma. Less-individualist cultures would scarcely recognize this as a sane or sensible goal, as their definitional parameters for health include the wellness of the family, greater community, and natural environment. Might the Western world learn something from this? Is it possible that what we need is less navel gazing, and more kinship—with humans and nonhumans alike?

Viewed through the lens of scientific materialism, psychedelics are chemical molecules that affect neurotransmitters mechanistically. In indigenous healing systems, however, these medicines are seen as *beings*. Journeyers often feel a presence: the mother (or grandmother) encountered in ayahuasca ceremonies, the *niños santos* ("holy children") of the Mazatec mushroom tradition, Grandfather Peyote (as the Wixárika call him), and countless other personifications. These substances are understood cross-culturally as discrete intelligences, often representing or connected with larger spiritual entities or deities.

As a result, journeyers in traditional settings have a reverential relationship with the medicine, often engaging in ceremonies of gratitude and reciprocity. In these traditions, shamans and healers are understood to be collaborating with the plants and fungi, seeing themselves as servants of a greater healing force, guardians of sacred knowledge. An equivalent orientation of humility and deep gratitude is often missing from modern approaches to psychedelics.

This reverential relationship to plant sacraments gets extended to the natural world as a whole. Plants and animals are understood to be relatives of humanity—which, of course, evolutionary theory confirms. As such, they make claims on the human community, and are deserving of respect and the freedom to live. The shaman, in many primary cultures, is not only a healer, but the one responsible for balancing the human and nonhuman worlds. Shamans utilize various "techniques of ecstasy" (Eliade, 1951/1964) to reach expanded states, communicating with the unseen on behalf of the human community, bringing back messages for the group about how to live in balance with the world around them.

On a planet rife with habitat destruction, resource depletion, and what some scientists are calling the "sixth mass extinction" (Kolbert, 2014), we appear to desperately need a reawakening to this wisdom: collectively remembering that the world and its inhabitants are alive, and *like us*, respecting the others with whom we share this world. Psychedelic experiences may be one of the surest avenues to this realization.

CUTTING THROUGH PSYCHEDELIC MATERIALISM

As psychedelic-assisted therapy becomes more widespread, we hope the field can move beyond its mundane goals. Chögyam Trungpa Rinpoche (1973) was among the first to recognize the danger of *spiritual materialism*, where one undertakes spiritual practice in order to feel better and succeed in a materialist culture. The psychedelic "industry" shows troubling signs of this trend, which we call *psychedelic materialism*. Journeys, we're told, afford us a chance to become better, more lovable, and more accomplished versions of who we've been. Perhaps a journey will unlock a vision for a new startup, or give us ideas for that book we've been meaning to write. Such attitudes grimly reflect our psychedelic materialism. But if we can cut through this distortion, and approach the medicine with humility, reverence, and a readiness to let go of the ego, what psychedelics will likely reveal is our basic goodness, our longing for connection, and our knowing that—though we're not special—we're OK, that we belong.

The psychedelic experience contains the seed of personal healing, yes, but also the possibility of transforming society. Rather than helping people adjust to what Abraham Maslow (1970) called the "psychopathology of the average" (p. 177), psychedelics open doors to deeper verities. If we as individuals can enter these doors and discover truer ways of being, then perhaps together we can form a new collective, one reflecting the wisdom of the old ways, bound to all of life in an ineradicable entanglement that is *home*.

CHAPTER 15

Completion . . . and Beyond

There is a coming home. A home base.
Psychedelics help you reconnect with home.
—ANN SHULGIN

We began this book with personal stories, moments when misadventures with psychedelics marred our psyches. We close the book with another set of stories—same people, but *very* different outcomes. Acknowledging the inherent danger of these drugs is essential, and we must exercise discernment around who is a good candidate for this work and how to best support them. That being said, we do have a personal stake in this. It was our firsthand experience of psychedelic-assisted therapy's transformative power that compelled us to write this book. We, too, have been on a journey. . . .

THE YOUNG MAN, NOW GROWN INTO MIDLIFE, FELT THE mushrooms start to kick in.

He had long since outgrown the revolutionary fervor of his youth, had ceased attacking the system and had chosen to become a healer. It was inward that his path of transformation had led him. The trauma of his bad trip long ago still flared up from time to time. He had the sense that if he reentered that same state of mind, after all the work he'd done, then maybe he could renegotiate the harrowing experience, and would at last be free.

He'd come to the office of a licensed psilocybin facilitator in Portland, Oregon—the first state in the nation to have legalized psilocybin-assisted therapy. The facilitator greeted him with a warm smile. They'd already done some work together to prepare for this day, and being in his presence again put the man at ease. The idea of taking mushrooms again raked his nerves, yes, but the guide was grounded, caring, and competent. The man drew a long breath, sighing with relief and curiosity.

The room was cozy and softly lit, with pillows and blankets everywhere, more like a living room than an office. The pale light of morning streamed through the double window. He squinted at the sunlight and it began to shimmer, the edges of the furniture melting like butter.

It was happening, then.

He closed his eyes. Long spirals of color whirled on the backs of his eyelids.

And his body! It glowed, crackled with electricity, radiating warmth. His muscles felt gooey and elastic, waves of formless relaxation rippling through him. The sensations were strange, but undeniably compelling.

As his body unfurled, so did his mind. Far-flung ideas began to knit together in a fluid synergy of disparate feelings and thoughts. Accompanying them was a cascade of mythic symbols, indelibly imbued with meaning too profound for words, all of it flowing through him.

He forced himself to breathe. He wasn't used to this sort of thing anymore. Decades had passed since he'd touched any kind of drug, even alcohol. He normally felt a kind of authorship over his thoughts and feelings, a sense of freely choosing. Well, that was out the window. He wasn't authoring any of this, and it was *a lot*. Each new emergence in his mind was a surprise, and this was beginning to concern him. He tried to remember his positive experiences in altered states, ones that had been life affirming: rituals and meditation retreats. He encouraged himself to let go, like his guide had told him.

Realizations began to take shape, patterns he recognized had been sewn throughout his lifespan, vaguely familiar, yet revelatory. He realized he had never truly felt loved, that he put up walls to keep people out, to keep them from hurting him. Now he saw that they also kept people from *seeing* him, from loving him. His mother had always relied on him for emotional stability—especially after his dad walked out on them—so he'd grown up convinced that relationships were transactional in nature, were about being there for someone else. If he ever felt appreciated, it was for something he *did* instead of who he *was*. And finally seeing this, it struck him as one of those pivotal moments when his life might never be the same.

Then, somehow, he was able to appreciate *himself*. His body sagged with relief as tears spilled from the corners of his eyes.

The man thought of the old cliché: "You can't love someone until you love yourself." But it knocked him down this time because he could see that it was *true*, and that he'd utterly failed to do it. Tears streamed down his face, the music in his headphones rising up and crashing down, changing in unison with his seismic shift in perspective. And it wasn't just that you couldn't love someone until you loved yourself, he now saw, you also couldn't truly *feel loved by another* without self-love, and all at once he understood why he'd never in his life felt truly loved. His shoulders shook with sobs, and he was grateful—so grateful for this journey, grateful to the mushrooms for handing him gifts he'd sought for as long as he could remember.

Then something changed. The music sounded louder, but he hadn't adjusted the volume. The visions seemed to speed up, blurring past him in a wild torrent of light and color. His body had no form at all. These thoughts, these images, these sensations, they were all so much and so strange, and this strangeness challenged his ability to stay present. It was getting out of control. A cold, creeping fear began to take hold of him, and the specter of insanity arose in his mind.

On some level he knew that if he hadn't gone crazy already, it was *extremely* unlikely to happen now. Secretly, though, he often gnawed over the possibility that he was a latent schizophrenic. No psychosis in his family, no history of a mental break—the facilitator would've screened him out of the treatment, had there been—but his years of panic attacks had made him fear he was destined for insanity, all of which had originated with that one bad mushroom trip as a teen.

The bad mushroom trip. That was why he'd come here in the first place—to renegotiate that horrific experience. Remembering his intention, he drew a long breath and resolved to sit with this feeling, experience it and see if it would pass. He shared none of this with his guide.

The facilitator looked him over and, determining that everything was fine, got up and went to the bathroom.

The very next moment a shockwave of anxiety tore through the man. His jaw clenched. His limbs seized with tension, nails digging into the couch like he was clinging to it for his very life. Suddenly he was right back where he'd started, decades ago: *alone and on mushrooms*. The precise conditions that had run his life off the rails as a kid.

"Why did I do this to myself?" he thought miserably. An ominous presence appeared just then. He could feel it looming over him, drawing closer. An image came into focus of the Indian

Ocean tsunami that had killed thousands. The massive black wave roared above him.

"Oh, God," he thought, "here it comes. This is it." The man saw himself as a tiny figure in front of that monstrous swell. He braced for impact, watching in mute dread as the soul-erasing darkness crested over him.

Then the wave broke. It crashed on top of him, subsuming him beneath the black waters. He was undone by it, erased from existence.

For a while there was nothing.

Slowly, though, he began to recognize that somehow, in some form, he was still there. The waters ebbed. The darkness receded. And he found that something within him was intact. It was tiny at first, just a little blip of light, but he could feel it—the aliveness in his body, his breath, the vital force animating him, and it was growing.

He was returning to coherence now, a sense of self gradually coming online. The man was stunned, grateful to realize he'd survived. No, he hadn't just survived—he had *prevailed*. He'd discovered his adamantine core, the indestructible center of himself, a light that could never be extinguished. He saw the possibility of inhabiting his body—and the world—in a different way, not in abstract theoretical terms but in a real sense, connected to his life force.

Gone was the familiar panic, the needling fear of madness. He thought of the coping strategies he'd developed in his youth to keep it under control: roving the city streets, asking people for the time every few minutes in a vain attempt to tamp it back down. This time, though, he hadn't tried to control the fear at all. He'd looked directly into it, seen it for what it was: insubstantial in its essence, wholly unthreatening. In trusting the medicine, and the container created by his facilitator, he had flowed with the process rather than against it, allowing it to show him the deeper aspects of his being. A chill ran down his spine, recognizing another one of those pivotal moments when his life might never be the same.

"I'm back," his guide said, closing the office door behind him. "How did things go?"

The man, grown from his youth but suddenly brimming with childlike glee, opened his eyes. A broad smile spread over his face. "Well," he slurred, "I guess I've got a story to tell you."

THE JUNGLE ENVELOPED HER LIKE A LIVING TAPESTRY, VIBRANT greens intertwining in a dance of shadow and light. Each leaf whispered secrets of healing, inviting her to shed the weight of her past. As she sank into the soft earth, her body felt heavy with generations of accumulated grief, her tears pouring forth as an offering to the ground beneath her. In this cathartic surrender, the soil absorbed her tears, a sacred exchange between her pain and its nurturing embrace.

This place felt achingly familiar, echoing with the primal wails of her ancestors. Their suffering harmonized with hers in a symphony of anguish that resonated above the canopy. Yet, a gentle presence emerged amid this sorrow—a warm, reassuring hand. The steady touch of her indigenous guide served as a soothing balm, his song wrapping around her, assuring her of safety. Her friends, each carrying their own burdens, sat beside her, anchoring her spirit in this moment of vulnerability.

As the tropical air whirled around her, she realized in that moment that she was transforming. After a lifetime of walking the rocky paths of therapy and introspection—a long journey marked by pain, intergenerational trauma, and cultural dissonance—she had finally come home to her own body. Home, she now saw, was not a literal place but a state of being. For too long she'd believed that home belonged to those with unbroken lineages, with firm roots. Through dance, movement practice, and creative expression, she had transformed her body into a sanctuary—however, over the years, she had drifted away from that sense of sacredness. Lost in the chaos of adulthood, the scars of trauma had obscured her knowing, distancing her from her true self.

She felt her guide's hand, warm and firm on her arm, his steadfast presence grounding her, anchoring her. His compassion radiated out toward her, and all at once she saw how different this place was from the office of the psychedelic therapist who'd scarred her as a youth. She sensed her guide's sincerity, his care rekindling her trust in the therapeutic connection.

She lay prone on the jungle floor, her heartbeat synchronizing with the earth's pulse, and its wisdom flowed into her, urging her to reclaim the trust she had lost. The medicine, the warmth of her companions, the presence of her guide, and the embrace of the jungle all came together and lifted the weight of her past. Her trauma began to dissolve, revealing something she thought she'd never find: a path of true healing. Memories flooded over her—dancing in the wheat fields as a child, back when she was still fluent in the language of joy, when her body had been a vessel of expression, alive with vibrant rhythm.

The remnants of trauma continued to lift, and she no longer had the urge to flee. She could simply be here, and breathe, and feel the full spectrum of her existence. Grief and healing coexisted within her, braided together like the massive tree roots overspreading the jungle floor. She was not alone, and never had been. She was part of something greater—a lineage of resilience and strength that transcended time.

This sacred space held her pain, yes, but also cradled her hope. She sensed a new possibility emerging, an invitation to rewrite her story, to honor both the weight of her past and the lightness of her spirit. Life force teemed all around her, beneath the canopy and beyond it, reminding her that healing is not linear; it ebbs and flows like the river winding through the underbrush.

As she sat there, tears mingling with the earth, she realized that she belonged here—in this jungle, in this world, and that her journey had led her here for a reason. Surrounded by nature, community, and a caring guide, her heart expanded, ready to meet the future with newfound trust in her body and its wisdom. The past no longer defined her but became part of a beautiful mosaic, one she was still creating. She felt the strength of her limbs, knowing she could finally stand tall, rooted in her own truth.

WE OFFER THESE STORIES AS EVIDENCE THAT TRANSFORMATION is possible, and as sources of hope. We know from direct experience that psychedelics can liberate human beings from outmoded patterns of mental and physical functioning: the limiting beliefs, emotional reactivity, bodily constriction, and existential numbness that keep us locked in maladaptive habits. They open doors to new discoveries and, potentially, a freedom never thought possible. We are grateful to have accessed this liberation in our own lives—and, if you are inspired to open this door for others, we hope this book can help you provide the best support possible.

Exercise: Walking Yourself Home

This exercise can be useful during the integration phase, a way of engaging the creative imagination to facilitate a sense of completion. It can also help prepare us for a next stage, or phase, of a larger healing journey.

1. Imagine a place where you feel most at home. This could be a natural setting, a dream location, or the place where you live. Visualize this place, seeing its contours and the way it feels like the place you belong.
2. Now, imagine that you are standing, seeing this place far away. Get a sense of this distance, and begin to close it, journeying in the direction of your home.
3. As you walk, highlight the milestones of your life's journey. Picture the landscape, seeing it filled with unique sights, strange visitors, magical moments, or traumatic memories.
4. Whatever you encounter, continue walking. Allow yourself to see, sense, and witness all that has transpired, staying present with each step. Feel your feet on the earth, noticing the rhythm of your breath as it flows in and out.
5. See your home again as you come nearer. As you walk, take in everything along your path. There's no need to grasp at anything, or to act—just keep walking.
6. When you arrive at your doorstep, pause and reflect on how far you've come.
7. Step inside your home and settle down. You have arrived; you are here.
8. What gifts have you brought with you? What is your home like now? Are you truly at home?

GROWING INTO MATURITY

Psychedelic-assisted therapy is an initiation into maturity. The seeker often arrives wanting knowledge, eager to release pain and receive comfort, perhaps looking for assurance that they are fundamentally worthy and really do belong on this earth.

But what they meet is a mystery. Psychedelic medicines have a plan beyond our human imagination or will. The journeyer is invited into uncertainty, and meets themselves in frightening and inspiring ways. Yet, as Shepard (1982) wrote, " . . . inherent in maturity [is] an acceptance of ambiguity" (p. 13). The therapist's ethical and compassionate guidance stewards this sacred alchemy.

Navigating hope and fear, without getting trapped in polarization, is essential for maturity. Learning to trust experience—both the sacred and the profane—allows for a realignment of basic assumptions. This shift enables a connection with what has been fractured or lost within.

The broken parts of ourselves are not inherently flawed—they just haven't been related to in the right way. With the help of psychedelics, we embrace and heal those fragmented aspects of our being. We attain true adulthood, or psychological maturity, an ability to gracefully bear the burden of ourselves, not just for our own benefit but in order to reimagine this culture. As Plotkin (2008) wrote, "All such adults are true artists, visionaries, and leaders, whether they live and work quietly in small arenas . . . or very publicly on grand stages. They are our most reliable agents of cultural change" (p. 8).

A central feature of maturity, of course, is humility. To experience psychedelic expansion is to meet a power greater than ourselves, discovering a world much larger than we'd imagined. This affords awe, a reckoning with how small we really are in the grand scheme of things. We begin to think of ourselves less.

CONCLUSION

Our aim is to make somatically informed psychedelic work available to as many people who want it—in as safe a way as possible. This requires taking a new approach to psychedelic-assisted therapy, one that is somatically informed and trauma sensitive, readying therapists to deepen the work and contain the journey.

As we've seen in this book, one needs to inhabit the body to live in the light of the mind. Our organism is a repository of wisdom, ready to guide us toward healing and reconnect us with the natural rhythms of existence. This work relies on the wisdom of the body, and also the wisdom of psychedelics themselves. These medicines have an intelligence all their own. With their help, we can learn to integrate the fragmented aspects of our being, not only for our own benefit but for the benefit of our world.

The psychedelic-assisted somatic therapist also embodies multiple roles—artist, visionary, leader—shaped by their unique journey toward full humanness. They engage their own inner work diligently, including their own journeys. This is a continuous path toward the full unfolding of the human person, undertaken with an attitude of reverence for the body, reverence for the medicine, and reverence for the inherent sacredness of all life.

REFERENCES

Aday, J. S., Davis, A. K., Mitzkovitz, C. M., Bloesch, E. K., & Davoli, C. C. (2021). Predicting reactions to psychedelic drugs: A systematic review of states and traits related to acute drug effects. *ACS Pharmacology and Translational Science, 4*(2), 424–435. https://doi.org/10.1021/acsptsci.1c00014

Aixalà, M. (2017, December 5). *Developing integration of visionary experiences: A future without integration.* Chacruna. https://chacruna.net/developing-integration-visionary

Aixalà, M. (2022). *Psychedelic integration.* Synergetic Press.

Algoe, S. B. (2012). Find, remind, and bind: The functions of gratitude in everyday relationships. *Social and Personality Psychology Compass, 6*(6), 455–469. https://doi.org/10.1111/j.1751-9004.2012.00439.x

American Association for Marriage and Family Therapy. (2015). *AAMFT code of ethics.* https://www.aamft.org/Legal_Ethics/Code_of_Ethics.aspx

American Psychedelic Practitioners Association. (2023). *Professional practice guidelines for psychedelic-assisted therapy practitioners.* https://www.appa-us.org/standards-and-guidelines/professionalpracticeguidelines

American Psychiatric Association. (2013). *Diagnostic and statistical manual of mental disorders* (5th ed.). https://doi.org/10.1176/appi.books.9780890425596

American Psychological Association. (2017). *Ethical principles of psychologists and code of conduct* (2002, amended effective June 1, 2010, and January 1, 2017). https://www.apa.org/ethics/code

American Psychological Association. (2023). *Stress in America: The impact of discrimination on mental health.* https://www.apa.org/news/press/releases/stress/2023/collective-trauma-recovery

Ardiel, E. L., & Rankin, C. H. (2010). The importance of touch in development. *Paediatrics and Child Health, 15*(3), 153–156. https://doi.org/10.1093/pch/15.3.153

Argyri, E. K., Evans, J., Luke, D., Michael, P., Michelle, K., Rohani-Shukla, C., Suseelan, S., Prideaux, E., McAlpine, R., Murphy-Beiner, A., & Robinson, O. (2024). Navigating groundlessness: An interview study on dealing with ontological shock and existential distress following psychedelic experiences. *SSRN Electronic Journal.* https://doi.org/10.2139/ssrn.4817368

Baggott, M. J., Coyle, J. R., Erowid, E., Erowid, F., & Robertson, L. C. (2011). Abnormal visual experiences in individuals with histories of hallucinogen use: A web-based questionnaire. *Drug and Alcohol Dependence, 114*(1), 61–67. https://doi.org/10.1016/j.drugalcdep.2010.09.006

Bandura, A. (1982). Self-efficacy mechanism in human agency. *American Psychologist, 37*(2), 122–147. https://doi.org/10.1037/0003-066X.37.2.122

Barstow, C. (2015). *Right use of power: The heart of ethics.* Many Realms.

Bathje, G. J., Majeski, E., & Kudowor, M. (2022). Psychedelic integration: An analysis of the concept and its practice. *Frontiers in Psychology, 13*, Article 824077. https://doi.org/10.3389/fpsyg.2022.824077

Berman, M. G., Jonides, J., & Kaplan, S. (2008). The cognitive benefits of interacting with nature. *Psychological Science, 19*(12), 1207–1212. https://doi.org/c97t5p

Bonny, H. L., & Pahnke, W. N. (1972). The use of music in psychedelic (LSD) psychotherapy. *Journal of Music Therapy, 9*(2), 64–87. https://doi.org/10.1093/jmt/9.2.64

Bratman, G. N., Hamilton, J. P., & Daily, G. C. (2012). The impacts of nature experience on human cognitive function and mental health. *Annals of the New York Academy of Sciences, 1249*(1), 118–136. https://doi.org/10.1111/j.1749-6632.2011.06400.x

Bratman, G. N., Olvera-Alvarez, H. A., & Gross, J. J. (2021). The affective benefits of nature exposure. *Social and Personality Psychology Compass, 15*(8), Article e12630. https://doi.org/10.1111/spc3.12630

Brom, D., Stokar, Y., Lawi, C., Nuriel-Porat, V., Ziv, Y., Lerner, K., & Ross, G. (2017). Somatic experiencing for posttraumatic stress disorder: A randomized controlled outcome study. *Journal of Traumatic Stress, 30*(3), 304–312. https://doi.org/10.1002/jts.22189

Brown, B. (2007). *I thought it was just me (but it isn't): Making the journey from "What will people think?" to "I am enough."* Avery.

Carbonaro, T. M., Bradstreet, M. P., Barrett, F. S., MacLean, K. A., Jesse, R., Johnson, M. W., & Griffiths, R. R. (2016). Survey study of challenging experiences after ingesting psilocybin mushrooms: Acute and enduring positive and negative consequences. *Journal of Psychopharmacology, 30*(12), 1268–1278. https://doi.org/10.1177/0269881116662634

Carhart-Harris, R. L., Bolstridge, M., Rucker, J., Day, C. M., Erritzoe, D., Kaelen, M., Bloomfield, M., Rickard, J. A., Forbes, B., Feilding, A., Taylor, D., Pilling, S., Curran, V. H., & Nutt, D. J. (2016). Psilocybin with psychological support for treatment-resistant depression: An open-label feasibility study. *Lancet Psychiatry, 3*(7), 619–627. https://doi.org/10.1016/s2215-0366(16)30065-7

Carhart-Harris, R. L., Chandaria, S., Erritzoe, D., Gazzaley, A., Girn, M., Kettner, H., Mediano, P., Nutt, D., Rosas, F., Roseman, L., Timmermann, C., Weiss, B., Zeifman, R., & Friston, K. (2023). Canalization and plasticity in psychopathology. *Neuropharmacology, 226*, Article 109398. https://doi.org/10.1016/j.neuropharm.2022.109398

Carhart-Harris, R. L., & Friston, K. J. (2019). REBUS and the anarchic brain: Toward a unified model of the brain action of psychedelics. *Pharmacological Reviews, 71*(3), 316–344. https://doi.org/10.1124/pr.118.017160

Carhart-Harris, R. L., Roseman, L., Bolstridge, M., Demetriou, L., Pannekoek, J. N., Wall, M. B., Tanner, M., Kaelen, M., McGonigle, J., Murphy, K., Leech, R., Curran, H. V., & Nutt, D. J. (2017). Psilocybin for treatment-resistant depression: fMRI-measured brain mechanisms. *Scientific Reports, 7*(1), Article 13187. https://doi.org/10.1038/s41598-017-13282-7Center for Cognitive Liberty and Ethics. (2003, February 7). *2C-B: A brief overview.* https://www.cognitiveliberty.org/ccle1/shulgin/adsarchive/2cb.htm

Charnetski, C. J., Riggers, S., & Brennan, F. X. (2004). Effect of petting a dog on immune system function. *Psychological Reports, 95*(3, Suppl. 1), 1087–1091. https://doi.org/10.2466/pr0.95.3f.1087-1091

Conde-Agudelo, A., & Díaz-Rossello, J. L. (2016). Kangaroo mother care to reduce morbidity and mortality in low birthweight infants. *Cochrane Database of Systematic Reviews, 2017*(2). https://doi.org/10.1002/14651858.cd002771.pub4

Conrad, E. (1997). *Life on land: The story of Continuum.* North Atlantic Books.

Cousin, L., Redwine, L., Bricker, C., Kip, K., & Buck, H. (2020). Effect of gratitude on cardiovascular health outcomes: A state-of-the-science review. *Journal of Positive Psychology, 16*(3), 348–355. https://doi.org/10.1080/17439760.2020.1716054

Creighton, L. (1906). *Life and letters of Mandell Creighton, D. D. Oxon. and Cam. sometime bishop of London.* Longmans, Green.

Cristóbal Cañadas, D., Parrón Carreño, T., Sánchez Borja, C., & Bonillo Perales, A. (2022). Benefits of kangaroo mother care on the physiological stress parameters of preterm infants and mothers in neonatal intensive care. *International Journal of Environmental Research and Public Health, 19*(12), Article 7183. https://doi.org/10.3390/ijerph19127183

Cuijpers, P., de Wit, L., Weitz, E., Andersson, G., & Huibers, M. J. H. (2015). The combination of psychotherapy and pharmacotherapy in the treatment of adult depression: A comprehensive meta-analysis. *Journal of Evidence-Based Psychotherapies, 15*(2), 147–168.

Damasio, A. R. (2003). *Looking for spinoza: Joy, sorrow and the feeling brain.* Heinemann.

Damasio, A. R. (2005). *Descartes' error: Emotion, reason, and the human brain.* Penguin.

Davidson, R. J., Kabat-Zinn, J., Schumacher, J., Rosenkranz, M., Muller, D., Santorelli, S. F., Urbanowski, F., Harrington, A., Bonus, K., & Sheridan, J. F. (2003). Alterations in brain and immune function produced by mindfulness meditation. *Psychosomatic Medicine, 65*(4), 564–570. https://doi.org/10.1097/01.psy.0000077505.67574.e3

Davis, A. K., Barrett, F. S., May, D. G., Cosimano, M. P., Sepeda, N. D., Johnson, M. W., Finan, P. H., & Griffiths, R. R. (2021). Effects of psilocybin-assisted therapy on major depressive disorder. *JAMA Psychiatry, 78*(5), 481–489. https://doi.org/10.1001/jamapsychiatry.2020.3285

Daws, R. E., Timmermann, C., Giribaldi, B., Sexton, J. D., Wall, M. B., Erritzoe, D., Roseman, L., Nutt, D., & Carhart-Harris, R. L. (2022). Increased global integration in the brain after psilocybin therapy for depression. *Nature Medicine, 28*(4), 844–851. https://doi.org/10.1038/s41591-022-01744-z

de Vos, C. M., Mason, N. L., & Kuypers, K. P. (2021). Psychedelics and neuroplasticity: A systematic review unraveling the biological underpinnings of psychedelics. *Frontiers in Psychiatry, 12*, Article 724606. https://doi.org/10.3389/fpsyt.2021.724606

Dias, B. G., & Ressler, K. J. (2013). Parental olfactory experience influences behavior and neural structure in subsequent generations. *Nature Neuroscience, 17*(1), 89–96. https://doi.org/10.1038/nn.3594

Dimberg, U., Thunberg, M., & Elmehed, K. (2000). Unconscious facial reactions to emotional facial expressions. *Psychological Science, 11*(1), 86–89. https://doi.org/10.1111/1467-9280.00221

Ekman, P. (2003). *Emotions revealed: Recognizing faces and feelings to improve communication and emotional life*. Times Books.

Eliade, M. (1964). *Shamanism: Archaic techniques of ecstasy* (W. R. Trask, Trans.). Bollingen Foundation. (Original work published 1951)

Ellis, H. (1898). Mescal: A new artificial paradise. *The Contemporary Review, 73*, 130–141.

Erritzoe, D., Barba, T., Greenway, K. T., Murphy, R., Martell, J., Giribaldi, B., Timmermann, C., Murphy-Beiner, A., Jones, M. B., Nutt, D. J., Weiss, B., & Carhart-Harris, R. L. (2024). Effect of psilocybin versus escitalopram on depression symptom severity in patients with moderate-to-severe major depressive disorder: Observational 6-month follow-up of a phase 2, double-blind, randomised, controlled trial. *eClinicalMedicine*, Article 102799. https://doi.org/10.1016/j.eclinm.2024.102799

Estrada, A. (1981). *María Sabina: Her life and chants* (H. Munn, Trans.). Ross-Erikson.

Evans, J., Robinson, O. C., Argyri, E. K., Suseelan, S., Murphy-Beiner, A., McAlpine, R., Luke, D., Michelle, K., & Prideaux, E. (2023). Extended difficulties following the use of psychedelic drugs: A mixed methods study. *PLoS One, 18*(10), Article e0293349. https://doi.org/10.1371/journal.pone.0293349

Fagetti, A., & Mercadillo, R. E. (2022). Experiences with sacred mushrooms and psilocybin in dialogue: Transdisciplinary interpretations of the "velada." *Anthropology of Consciousness, 33*(2), 385–411. https://doi.org/10.1111/anoc.12163

Feldman, R., Rosenthal, Z., & Eidelman, A. I. (2010). Maternal-preterm skin-to-skin contact enhances child physiologic organization and cognitive control across the first 10 years of life. *Biological Psychiatry, 75*(1), 56–64. https://doi.org/10.1016/j.biopsych.2013.08.012

Field, T. M. (2001). *Touch*. MIT Press.

Field, T. M., Schanberg, S. M., Scafidi, F., Bauer, C. R., Vega-Lahr, N., Garcia, R., Nystrom, J., & Kuhn, C. M. (1986). Tactile/kinesthetic stimulation effects on preterm neonates. *Pediatrics, 77*(5), 654–658. https://doi.org/10.1542/peds.77.5.654

Francis, D. D., & Kuhar, M. J. (2008). Frequency of maternal licking and grooming correlates negatively with vulnerability to cocaine and alcohol use in rats. *Pharmacology Biochemistry and Behavior, 90*(3), 497–500. https://doi.org/10.1016/j.pbb.2008.04.012

Freud, S. (1913). *The interpretation of dreams* (A. A. Brill, Trans.). Macmillan. (Original work published 1899)

Garakani, A., Alexander, J. L., Sumner, C. R., Pine, J. H., Gross, L. S., Raison, C. L., Aaronson, S. T., & Baron, D. A. (2023). Psychedelics, with a focus on psilocybin: Issues for the clinician. *Journal of Psychiatric Practice, 29*(5), 345–353. https://doi.org/10.1097/pra.0000000000000729

Geltner, P. (2012). *Emotional communication: Countertransference analysis and the use of feeling in psychoanalytic technique*. Routledge. https://doi.org/10.4324/9780203081280

Gendlin, E. T. (1981). *Focusing.* Bantam Books.

Goldstein, A. N., & Walker, M. P. (2014). The role of sleep in emotional brain function. *Annual Review of Clinical Psychology, 10*(1), 679–708. https://doi.org/10.1146/ann urev-clinpsy-032813-153716

Gonzalez, D., Cantillo, J., Perez, I., Carvalho, M., Aronovich, A., Farre, M., Feilding, A., Obiols, J. E., & Bouso, J. C. (2021). The Shipibo ceremonial use of ayahuasca to promote well-being: An observational study. *Frontiers in Pharmacology, 12.* https://doi.org/10.3389/fphar.2021.623923

Governor Shafer calls LSD blindings a hoax; Story of six students who stared at sun is laid to a Pennsylvania official. (1968, January 19). *The New York Times.*

Griffiths, R. R., Johnson, M. W., Carducci, M. A., Umbricht, A., Richards, W. A., Richards, B. D., Cosimano, M. P., & Klinedinst, M. A. (2016). Psilocybin produces substantial and sustained decreases in depression and anxiety in patients with life-threatening cancer: A randomized double-blind trial. *Journal of Psychopharmacology, 30*(12), 1181–1197. https://doi.org/10.1177/0269881116675513

Griffiths, R. R., Johnson, M. W., Richards, W. A., Richards, B. D., McCann, U., & Jesse, R. (2011). Psilocybin occasioned mystical-type experiences: Immediate and persisting dose-related effects. *Psychopharmacology, 218*(4), 649–665. https://doi.org/10.1007/s00213-011-2358-5

Griffiths, R. R., Richards, W. A,, Johnson, M. W., McCann, U. D., & Jesse, R. (2008). Mystical-type experiences occasioned by psilocybin mediate the attribution of personal meaning and spiritual significance 14 months later. *Journal of Psychopharmacology, 22*(6), 621–632. https://doi.org/10.1177/0269881108094300Griffiths, R. R., Richards, W. A., McCann, U., & Jesse, R. (2006). Psilocybin can occasion mystical-type experiences having substantial and sustained personal meaning and spiritual significance. *Psychopharmacology, 187*(3), 268–283. https://doi.org/10.1007/s00213-006-0457-5Grinspoon, L., & Bakalar, J. B. (1979). *Psychedelic drugs reconsidered.* Basic Books.

Grof, S. (1980). *LSD psychotherapy.* Hunter House.

Grof, S. (2006). *When the impossible happens: Adventures in non-ordinary realities.* Sounds True.

Grof, S., & Grof, C. (2023). *Holotropic breathwork: A new approach to self-exploration and therapy* (2nd ed.). State University of New York Press.

Gutkowska, J., & Jankowski, M. (2011). Oxytocin revisited: Its role in cardiovascular regulation. *Journal of Neuroendocrinology, 24*(4), 599–608. https://doi.org/10.1111/j.1365-2826.2011.02235.x

H. Con. Res. 331—100th Congress. (1988). A concurrent resolution to acknowledge the contribution of the Iroquois Confederacy of Nations to the development of the United States Constitution and to reaffirm the continuing government-to-government relationship between Indian tribes and the United States established in the Constitution. https://www.congress.gov/bill/100th-congress/house-concurrent-resolution/331

Haines, S. K. (2019). *The politics of trauma: Somatics, healing, and social justice.* North Atlantic Books.

Halpern, J. H., Lerner, A. G., & Passie, T. (2018). A review of hallucinogen persisting perception disorder (HPPD) and an exploratory study of subjects claiming symptoms of HPPD. In A. L. Halberstadt, F. X. Vollenweider, & D. E. Nichols (Eds.), *Behavioral neurobiology of psychedelic drugs* (pp. 333–360). Springer. https://doi.org/10.1007/7854_2016_457

Hartogsohn, I. (2017). Constructing drug effects: A history of set and setting. *Drug Science, Policy and Law, 3.* https://doi.org/10.1177/2050324516683325

Hartogsohn, I. (2020). *American trip: Set, setting, and the psychedelic experience in the twentieth century.* MIT Press.

Hassan, A., & Deshun, Z. (2023). Promoting adult health: The neurophysiological benefits of watering plants and engaging in mental tasks within designed environments. *BMC Psychology, 11*(1), Article 310. https://doi.org/10.1186/s40359-023-01362-5

Healy, D. (1997). *The antidepressant era.* Harvard University Press.

Hebb, D. O. (1949). *The organization of behavior: A neuropsychological theory.* Wiley.

Henrich, J., Heine, S. J., & Norenzayan, A. (2010). The weirdest people in the world? *Behavioral and Brain Sciences, 33,* 61–83. https://doi.org/10.1017/s0140525x0999152x

Herbert, F. (2003). *Dune.* Penguin.

Hofmann, A. (1980). *LSD, my problem child* (J. Ott, Trans.). McGraw-Hill.

Holze, F., Vizeli, P., Ley, L., Müller, F., Dolder, P., Stocker, M., Duthaler, U., Varghese, N., Eckert, A., Borgwardt, S., & Liechti, M. E. (2020). Acute dose-dependent effects of lysergic acid diethylamide in a double-blind placebo-controlled study in healthy subjects. *Neuropsychopharmacology, 46*(3), 537–544. https://doi.org/10.1038/s41386-020-00883-6

Hölzel, B. K., Carmody, J., Vangel, M., Congleton, C., Yerramsetti, S. M., Gard, T., & Lazar, S. W. (2011). Mindfulness practice leads to increases in regional brain gray matter density. *Psychiatry Research: Neuroimaging, 191*(1), 36–43. https://doi.org/10.1016/j.pscychresns.2010.08.006

Hunter, M. R., Gillespie, B. W., & Chen, S. Y.-P. (2019). Urban nature experiences reduce stress in the context of daily life based on salivary biomarkers. *Frontiers in Psychology, 10.* https://doi.org/10.3389%2Ffpsyg.2019.00722

Institute of Medicine. (2002). *Unequal treatment: Confronting racial and ethnic disparities in health care.* National Academies Press.

Jarczok, M. N., Weimer, K., Braun, C., Williams, D. P., Thayer, J. F., Gündel, H. O., & Balint, E. M. (2022). Heart rate variability in the prediction of mortality: A systematic review and meta-analysis of healthy and patient populations. *Neuroscience and Biobehavioral Reviews, 143,* Article 104907. https://doi.org/10.1016/j.neubiorev.2022.104907

Johansen, P.-Ø., & Krebs, T. S. (2015). Psychedelics not linked to mental health problems or suicidal behavior: A population study. *Journal of Psychopharmacology, 29*(3), 270–279. https://doi.org/10.1177/0269881114568039

Johanson, G. (2015). Hakomi principles and a systems approach to psychotherapy. In H. Weiss, G. Johanson, & L. Monda (Eds.), *Hakomi mindfulness-centered somatic psychotherapy* (pp. 41–57). Norton.

Johanson, G., & Kurtz, R. (1991). *Grace unfolding: Psychotherapy in the spirit of the Tao-te-ching.* Bell Tower.

Jones, J. M. (2021, March 29). *U.S. church membership falls below majority for first time*. Gallup. https://news.gallup.com/poll/341963/church-membership-falls-below-majority-first-time.aspx

Jung, C. G. (1969). *The collected works of C. G. Jung, Volume 9 (Part 2)*. (G. Adler & R. F. C. Hull, Eds.). Princeton University Press. (Original work published 1951) https://doi.org/10.1515/9781400851058

Jung, C. G. (1970). The meaning of psychology for modern man. In G. Adler & R. F. C. Hull (Eds.), *The collected works of C. G. Jung: Vol. 10. Civilization in transition* (2nd ed., pp. 134–156). Princeton University Press. (Original work published 1934) https://doi.org/10.1515/9781400850976.134

Kaelen, M., Giribaldi, B., Raine, J., Evans, L., Timmerman, C., Rodriguez, N., Roseman, L., Feilding, A., Nutt, D., & Carhart-Harris, R. L. (2018). The hidden therapist: Evidence for a central role of music in psychedelic therapy. *Psychopharmacology, 235*(2), 505–519. https://doi.org/10.1007%2Fs00213-017-4820-5

Kaimal, G., Ray, K., & Muniz, J. (2016). Reduction of cortisol levels and participants' responses following art making. *Art Therapy, 33*(2), 74–80. https://doi.org/10.1080/07421656.2016.1166832

Kearney, B. E., Terpou, B. A., Densmore, M., Shaw, S. B., Théberge, J., Jetly, R., McKinnon, M. C., & Lanius, R. A. (2023). How the body remembers: Examining the default mode and sensorimotor networks during moral injury autobiographical memory retrieval in PTSD. *NeuroImage: Clinical, 38*, Article 103426. https://doi.org/10.1016/j.nicl.2023.103426

Keltner, D. (2023). *Awe: The new science of everyday wonder and how it can transform your life*. Penguin.

Kettner, H., Gandy, S., Haijen, E. C., & Carhart-Harris, R. L. (2019). From egoism to ecoism: Psychedelics increase nature relatedness in a state-mediated and context-dependent manner. *International Journal of Environmental Research and Public Health, 16*(24), Article 5147. https://doi.org/10.3390/ijerph16245147

Kirsch, I., & Sapirstein, G. (1998). Listening to Prozac but hearing placebo: A meta-analysis of antidepressant medication. *Prevention and Treatment, 1*(2), Article 2a. https://doi.org/10.1037/1522-3736.1.1.12a

Koffel, E., Khawaja, I. S., & Germain, A. (2016). Sleep disturbances in posttraumatic stress disorder: Updated review and implications for treatment. *Psychiatric Annals, 46*(3), 173–176. https://doi.org/10.3928/00485713-20160125-01

Kolbert, E. (2014). *The sixth extinction: An unnatural history*. Holt.

Kounenou, K., Kalamatianos, A., Nikoltsiou, P., & Kourmousi, N. (2023). The interplay among empathy, vicarious trauma, and burnout in Greek mental health practitioners. *International Journal of Environmental Research and Public Health, 20*(4). https://doi.org/10.3390/ijerph20043503

Kourtzi, Z., & Connor, C. E. (2011). Neural representations for object perception: Structure, category, and adaptive coding. *Annual Review of Neuroscience, 34*, 45–67. https://doi.org/10.1146/annurev-neuro-060909-153218

Krediet, E., Bostoen, T., Breeksema, J., van Schagen, A., Passie, T., & Vermetten, E. (2020).

Reviewing the potential of psychedelics for the treatment of PTSD. *International Journal of Neuropsychopharmacology, 23*(6), 385–400. https://doi.org/10.1093/ijnp/pyaa018

Kurtz, R. (2015). *Body-centered psychotherapy: The Hakomi method.* LifeRhythm.

Leary, T., Metzner, R., & Alpert, R. (1992). *The psychedelic experience: A manual based on the Tibetan book of the dead.* Citadel Press.

Lee, M. A., & Shlain, B. (1992). *Acid dreams: The complete social history of LSD: The CIA, the sixties, and beyond.* Grove Press.

Levine, P. A. (1997). *Waking the tiger: Healing trauma through the body.* North Atlantic Books.

Levine, P. A. (2010). *In an unspoken voice: How the body releases trauma and restores goodness.* North Atlantic Books.

Levine, P. A. (2015). *Trauma and memory: Brain and body in a search for the living past: A practical guide for understanding and working with traumatic memory.* North Atlantic Books.

Liu, D., Diorio, J., Tannenbaum, B., Caldji, C., Francis, D., Freedman, A., Sharma, S., Pearson, D., Plotsky, P. M., & Meaney, M. J. (1997). Maternal care, hippocampal glucocorticoid receptors, and hypothalamic–pituitary–adrenal responses to stress. *Science, 277*(5332), 1659–1662. https://doi.org/10.1126/science.277.5332.1659

Lorenz, E. (1972, December 26–31). *Predictability: Does the flap of a butterfly's wing in Brazil set off a tornado in Texas?* [Paper presentation]. American Association for the Advancement of Science Annual Meeting, Washington, DC.

Luoma, J. (2023, July 17). *Touch Outcomes Measurement Inventory* (TOMI). OSF. https://osf.io/85nec

Lüönd, A. M., Wolfensberger, L., Wingenbach, T. S. H., Schnyder, U., Weilenmann, S., & Pfaltz, M. C. (2022). Don't get too close to me: Depressed and non-depressed survivors of child maltreatment prefer larger comfortable interpersonal distances towards strangers. *European Journal of Psychotraumatology, 13*(1), Article 2066457. https://doi.org/10.1080/20008198.2022.2066457

Magsamen, S. (2019). Your brain on art: The case for neuroaesthetics. *Cerebrum 2019*, 1–20. https://www.ncbi.nlm.nih.gov/pmc/articles/PMC7075503

Maslow, A. H. (1970). *Motivation and personality.* Harper & Row.

Maté, G. (2024, July 25). *Trauma.* https://drgabormate.com/trauma

McKenna, T. (1992). *Food of the gods: The search for the original tree of knowledge.* Bantam Books.

McLynn, F. (2014). *Carl Gustav Jung: A biography.* St. Martin's Press.

Meaney, M. J., & Szyf, M. (2005). Environmental programming of stress responses through DNA methylation: Life at the interface between a dynamic environment and a fixed genome. *Dialogues in Clinical Neuroscience, 7*(2), 103–123. https://doi.org/10.31887/dcns.2005.7.2/mmeaney

Mehrabian, A. (1971). *Silent messages.* Wadsworth.

Metzner, R. (2015). *Allies for awakening: Guidelines for productive and safe experiences with entheogens.* Regent Press.

Milner, A. D., & Goodale, M. A. (2008). Two visual systems re-viewed. *Neuropsychologia, 46*(3), 774–785. https://doi.org/10.1016/j.neuropsychologia.2007.10.005

Mitchell, J. M., Bogenschutz, M., Lilienstein, A., Harrison, C., Kleiman, S., Parker-Guilbert, K., Ot'alora, G. M., Garas, W., Paleos, C., Gorman, I., Nicholas, C., Mithoefer, M.,

Carlin, S., Poulter, B., Mithoefer, A., Quevedo, S., Wells, G., Klaire, S. S., van der Kolk, B., . . . Doblin, R. (2021). MDMA-assisted therapy for severe PTSD: A randomized, double-blind, placebo-controlled phase 3 study. *Nature Medicine, 27*(6), 1025–1033. https://doi.org/10.1038/s41591-021-01336-3

Mitchell, J. M., Ot'alora, G. M., van der Kolk, B., Shannon, S., Bogenschutz, M., Gelfand, Y., Paleos, C., Nicholas, C. R., Quevedo, S., Balliett, B., Hamilton, S., Mithoefer, M., Kleiman, S., Parker-Guilbert, K., Tzarfaty, K., Harrison, C., de Boer, A., Doblin, R., & Yazar-Klosinski, B. (2023). MDMA-assisted therapy for moderate to severe PTSD: A randomized, placebo-controlled phase 3 trial. *Nature Medicine, 29*(10), 2473–2480. https://doi.org/10.1038/s41591-023-02565-4

Mithoefer, M. C. (2016). *A manual for MDMA-assisted psychotherapy in the treatment of posttraumatic stress disorder.* Multidisciplinary Association for Psychedelic Studies. https://s3-us-west-1.amazonaws.com/mapscontent/research-archive/mdma/MDMAAssistedPsychotherapyTreatmentManualVersion+8_25May16_Formatted.pdf

Mithoefer, M. C., Mithoefer, A. T., Feduccia, A. A., Jerome, L., Wagner, M., Wymer, J., Holland, J., Hamilton, S., Yazar-Klosinski, B., Emerson, A., & Doblin, R. (2018). 3,4-methylenedioxymethamphetamine (MDMA)-assisted psychotherapy for posttraumatic stress disorder in military veterans, firefighters, and police officers: A randomised, double-blind, dose-response, phase 2 clinical trial. *The Lancet Psychiatry, 5*(6), 486–497. https://doi.org/10.1016/s2215-0366(18)30135-4

Mithoefer, M. C., Wagner, M. T., Mithoefer, A. T., Jerome, L., & Doblin, R. (2011). The safety and efficacy of ±3,4-methylenedioxymethamphetamine-assisted psychotherapy in subjects with chronic, treatment-resistant posttraumatic stress disorder: The first randomized controlled pilot study. *Journal of Psychopharmacology, 25*(4), 439–452. https://doi.org/10.1177/0269881110378371

Monroy, M., & Keltner, D. (2022). Awe as a pathway to mental and physical health. *Perspectives on Psychological Science, 18*(2), 309–320. https://doi.org/10.1177/17456916221094856

Morris, H., & Smith, A. (2013, May 16). The last interview with Alexander Shulgin. *Vice.* https://www.vice.com/en/article/the-last-interview-with-alexander-shulgin

Morris, J., Friston, K. J., Büchel, C., Frith, C. D., Young, A. W., Calder, A. J., & Dolan, R. J. (1998). A neuromodulatory role for the human amygdala in processing emotional facial expressions. *Brain, 121*(1), 47–57. https://doi.org/10.1093/brain/121.1.47

Morris, S. M. (2010). Achieving collective coherence: Group effects on heart rate variability coherence and heart rhythm synchronization. *Alternative Therapies in Health and Medicine, 16*(4), 62–72. https://www.heartmath.org/assets/uploads/2015/01/achieving-collective-coherence.pdf

Müller, F., Kraus, E., Holze, F., Becker, A., Ley, L., Schmid, Y., Vizeli, P., Liechti, M. E., & Borgwardt, S. (2022). Flashback phenomena after administration of LSD and psilocybin in controlled studies with healthy participants. *Psychopharmacology, 239*(6), 1933–1943. https://doi.org/10.1007/s00213-022-06066-z

Multidisciplinary Association for Psychedelic Studies. (2021). *MAPS code of ethics for psychedelic psychotherapy* (Version 4). https://maps.org/wp-content/uploads/2022/06

/MAPS_Psychedelic_Assisted_Psychotherapy_Code_of_Ethics_V4_22_June_2022_Final.pdf

Mustafa, R. A., McQueen, B., Nikitin, D., Nhan, E., Zemplenyi, A., DiStefano, M. J., Kayali, Y., Richardson, M., & Rind, D. M. (2024). *Midomafetamine-assisted psychotherapy for post-traumatic stress disorder* [Final evidence report]. Institute for Clinical and Economic Review. https://icer.org/wp-content/uploads/2024/06/PTSD_Final-Report_For-Publication_06272024.pdf

Nardou, R., Lewis, E. M., Rothhaas, R., Xu, R., Yang, A., Boyden, E., & Dölen, G. (2019). Oxytocin-dependent reopening of a social reward learning critical period with MDMA. *Nature, 569*(7754), 116–120. https://doi.org/10.1038/s41586-019-1075-9

National Center for PTSD. (2023, February 3). *How common is PTSD in adults?* U.S. Department of Veterans Affairs. https://www.ptsd.va.gov/understand/common/common_adults.asp

Ogden, P., Minton, K., & Pain, C. (2006). *Trauma and the body: A sensorimotor approach to psychotherapy*. Norton.

O'Neill, T. (2019). *Chaos: Charles Manson, the CIA, and the secret history of the sixties*. Little, Brown.

Oregon Health Authority. (2022). *Ethical principles/code of conduct for psilocybin facilitators*. https://www.oregon.gov/oha/PH/PREVENTIONWELLNESS/Documents/Ethical%20Principles-Code%20of%20Conduct%20for%20Jan%206%20Meeting%201-2-2022.pdf

Oregon Health Authority. (2024a). *Facilitator conduct*. Oregon Administrative Rules, OAR 333-333-5120. https://secure.sos.state.or.us/oard/viewSingleRule.action?ruleVrsnRsn=309289

Oregon Health Authority. (2024b). *Social equity plans*. Oregon Administrative Rules, OAR 333-333-4020. https://secure.sos.state.or.us/oard/viewSingleRule.action?ruleVrsnRsn=309242

Parkin, A. J., Reid, T. K., & Russo, R. (1990). On the differential nature of implicit and explicit memory. *Memory and Cognition, 18*(5), 507–514. https://doi.org/10.3758/bf03198483

Passie, T., Seifert, J., Schneider, U., & Emrich, H. M. (2002). The pharmacology of psilocybin. *Addiction Biology, 7*(4), 357–364. https://doi.org/10.1080/1355621021000005937

Pavlov, I. P. (1927). *Conditioned reflexes: An investigation of the physiological activity of the cerebral cortex* (G. V. Anrep, Ed. & Trans.). Oxford University Press.

Perls, F. S., Hefferline, R. F., & Goodman, P. (1951). *Gestalt therapy: Excitement and growth in the human personality*. Delta.

Phelps, J. (2017). Developing guidelines and competencies for the training of psychedelic therapists. *Journal of Humanistic Psychology, 57*(5), 450–487. https://doi.org/10.1177/0022167817711304

Plotkin, B. (2008). *Nature and the human soul*. New World Library.

Pollan, M. (2018). *How to change your mind: What the new science of psychedelics teaches us about consciousness, dying, addiction, depression, and transcendence*. Penguin.

Porges, S. W. (2011). *The polyvagal theory: Neurophysiological foundations of emotions, attachment, communication, and self-regulation*. Norton.

Porges, S. W. (2022). Polyvagal theory: A science of safety. *Frontiers in Integrative Neuroscience, 16,* Article 871227. https://doi.org/10.3389/fnint.2022.871227

Putnam, R. D. (2020). *Bowling alone: The collapse and revival of American community.* Simon & Schuster.

Ramesh, A., Nayak, T., Beestrum, M., Quer, G., & Pandit, J. (2023). Heart rate variability in psychiatric disorders: A systematic review. *Neuropsychiatric Disease and Treatment, Volume 19,* 2217–2239. https://doi.org/10.2147/ndt.s429592

Reiner, R. (Director). (1984). *This is spinal tap* [Film]. Embassy Pictures.

Richards, W. A. (2015). *Sacred knowledge: Psychedelics and religious experiences.* Columbia University Press.

Robinson, C., Fonseca, A., Diejomaoh, E., D'Souza, R., Schatman, M., Orhurhu, V., & Emerick, T. (2024). Scoping review: The role of psychedelics in the management of chronic pain. *Journal of Pain Research, 17,* 965–973. https://doi.org/10.2147/jpr.s439348

Rogers, C. (2012). *On becoming a person: A therapist's view of psychotherapy.* Houghton Mifflin.

Roseman, L., Nutt, D. J., & Carhart-Harris, R. L. (2018). Quality of acute psychedelic experience predicts therapeutic efficacy of psilocybin for treatment-resistant depression. *Frontiers in Pharmacology, 8.* https://doi.org/10.3389/fphar.2017.00974

Rothschild, B. (2000). *The body remembers: The psychophysiology of trauma and trauma treatment.* Norton.

Rotter, J. B. (1966). Generalized expectancies for internal versus external control of reinforcement. *Psychological Monographs: General and Applied, 80*(1), 1–28. https://doi.org/10.1037/h0092976

Schindler, E. A. D., Sewell, R. A., Gottschalk, C. H., Flynn, L. T., Zhu, Y., Pittman, B. P., Cozzi, N. V., & D'Souza, D. C. (2024). Psilocybin pulse regimen reduces cluster headache attack frequency in the blinded extension phase of a randomized controlled trial. *Journal of the Neurological Sciences, 460,* Article 122993. https://doi.org/10.1016/j.jns.2024.122993

Schlag, A. K., Aday, J., Salam, I., Neill, J. C., & Nutt, D. J. (2022). Adverse effects of psychedelics: From anecdotes and misinformation to systematic science. *Journal of Psychopharmacology, 36*(3), 258–272. https://doi.org/10.1177/02698811211069100

Schouten, K. A., de Niet, G. J., Knipscheer, J. W., Kleber, R. J., & Hutschemaekers, G. J. (2014). The effectiveness of art therapy in the treatment of traumatized adults. *Trauma, Violence, & Abuse, 16*(2), 220–228. https://doi.org/10.1177/1524838014555032

Selver, C., & Brooks, C. V. W. (2007). *Reclaiming vitality and presence: Sensory awareness as a practice for life* (R. Lowe & S. Laeng-Gilliatt, Eds.). North Atlantic Books.

Shepard, P. (1982). *Nature and madness.* Sierra Club Books.

Shukla, A., Choudhari, S. G., Gaidhane, A. M., & Quazi Syed, Z. (2022). Role of art therapy in the promotion of mental health: A critical review. *Cureus, 14*(8), Article e28026. https://doi.org/10.7759%2Fcureus.28026

Spitz, R. A. (1945). Hospitalism: An inquiry into the genesis of psychiatric conditions in early childhood. *The Psychoanalytic Study of the Child, 1*(1), 53–74. https://doi.org/10.1080/00797308.1945.11823126

Starhawk. (1989). *Truth or dare: Encounters with power, authority, and mystery.* Harper Collins.

Stolaroff, M. J. (2004). *The secret chief revealed*. Multidisciplinary Association for Psychedelic Studies.

Sweeney, M. M., Nayak, S., Hurwitz, E. S., Mitchell, L. N., Swift, T. C., & Griffiths, R. R. (2022). Comparison of psychedelic and near-death or other non-ordinary experiences in changing attitudes about death and dying. *PLoS One, 17*(8), Article e0271926. https://doi.org/10.1371/journal.pone.0271926

Taylor, A. G., Goehler, L. E., Galper, D. I., Innes, K. E., & Bourguignon, C. (2010). Top-down and bottom-up mechanisms in mind–body medicine: Development of an integrative framework for psychophysiological research. *Explore, 6*(1), 29–41. https://doi.org/10.1016/j.explore.2009.10.004

Taylor, K. (2017). *The ethics of caring: Finding right relationship with clients for profound, transformative work in our professional healing relationships*. Hanford Mead.

Thal, S. B., Wieberneit, M., Sharbanee, J. M., Skeffington, P. M., Bruno, R., Wenge, T., & Bright, S. J. (2023). Dosing and therapeutic conduct in administration sessions in substance-assisted psychotherapy: A systematized review. *Journal of Humanistic Psychology, 0*(0). https://doi.org/10.1177/00221678231168516

Tiwari, R., Kumar, R., Malik, S., Raj, T., & Kumar, P. (2021). Analysis of heart rate variability and implication of different factors on heart rate variability. *Current Cardiology Reviews, 17*(5), e160721189770. https://doi.org/10.2174/1573403x16999201231203854

Traynor, J. M., Roberts, D. E., Ross, S., Zeifman, R., & Choi-Kain, L. (2022). MDMA-assisted psychotherapy for borderline personality disorder. *Focus, 20*(4), 358–367. https://doi.org/10.1176/appi.focus.20220056

Tronick, E. Z. (2007). *The neurobehavioral and social–emotional development of infants and children*. Norton.

Trungpa, C. (1973). *Cutting through spiritual materialism*. Shambhala.

Trungpa, C. (1984). *Shambhala: The sacred path of the warrior*. Shambhala.

Vaid, G., & Walker, B. (2022). Psychedelic psychotherapy: Building wholeness through connection. *Global Advances in Integrative Medicine and Health, 11*. https://doi.org/10.1177/2164957X221081113

van der Meer, P. B., Fuentes, J. J., Kaptein, A. A., Schoones, J. W., de Waal, M. M., Goudriaan, A. E., Kramers, K., Schellekens, A., Somers, M., Bossong, M. G., & Batalla, A. (2023). Therapeutic effect of psilocybin in addiction: A systematic review. *Frontiers in Psychiatry, 14*. https://doi.org/10.3389/fpsyt.2023.1134454

Van Essen, D. C. (2003). Organization of visual areas in macaque and human cerebral cortex. In L. M. Chalupa & J. S. Werner (Eds.), *The visual neurosciences* (pp. 507–522). MIT Press.

Wasson, R. G. (1957, May 13). Seeking the magic mushroom. *Life, 42*(19), 100–120.

Welwood, J. (2000). *Toward a psychology of awakening: Buddhism, psychotherapy, and the path of personal and spiritual transformation*. Shambhala.

Wheeler, M., Cooper, N. R., Andrews, L., Hacker Hughes, J., Juanchich, M., Rakow, T., & Orbell, S. (2020). Outdoor recreational activity experiences improve psychological well-being of military veterans with post-traumatic stress disorder: Positive find-

ings from a pilot study and a randomised controlled trial. *PLoS One, 15*(11), Article e0241763. https://doi.org/10.1371/journal.pone.0241763
Willis, J., & Todorov, A. (2006). First impressions: Making up your mind after a 100-ms exposure to a face. *Psychological Science, 17*(7), 592–598. https://doi.org/10.1111/j.1467-9280.2006.01750.x
Winkelman, M. J. (2021). The evolved psychology of psychedelic set and setting: Inferences regarding the roles of shamanism and entheogenic experiences. *Frontiers in Psychology, 12*. https://doi.org/10.3389/fphar.2021.619890
Winnicott, D. W. (1965). *The maturational processes and the facilitating environment: Studies in the theory of emotional development*. International Universities Press.
Wood, A. M., Froh, J. J., & Geraghty, A. W. A. (2010). Gratitude and well-being: A review and theoretical integration. *Clinical Psychology Review, 30*(7), 890–905. https://doi.org/10.1016/j.cpr.2010.03.005
Wood, A. M., Joseph, S., Lloyd, J., & Atkins, S. (2009). Gratitude influences sleep through the mechanism of pre-sleep cognitions. *Journal of Psychosomatic Research, 66*(1), 43–48. https://doi.org/10.1016/j.jpsychores.2008.09.002Yehuda, R., & Lehrner, A. (2018). Intergenerational transmission of trauma effects: Putative role of epigenetic mechanisms. *World Psychiatry, 17*(3), 243–257. https://doi.org/10.1002/wps.20568
Yu, C., Yang, F., Yang, S., Tseng, P., Stubbs, B., Yeh, T., Hsu, C., Li, D., & Liang, C. (2021). Psilocybin for end-of-life anxiety symptoms: A systematic review and meta-analysis. *Psychiatry Investigation, 18*(10), 958–967. https://doi.org/10.30773/pi.2021.0209
Zaretsky, T. G., Jagodnik, K. M., Barsic, R., Antonio, J. H., Bonanno, P. A., MacLeod, C., Pierce, C., Carney, H., Morrison, M. T., Saylor, C., Danias, G., Lepow, L., & Yehuda, R. (2024). The psychedelic future of post-traumatic stress disorder treatment. *Current Neuropharmacology, 22*(4), 636–735. https://doi.org/10.2174/1570159X22666231027111147
Zayan, U., Da Prato, L. C., Muscatelli, F., & Matarazzo, V. (2023). Modulation of the thermosensory system by oxytocin. *Frontiers in Molecular Neuroscience, 15*. https://doi.org/10.3389/fnmol.2022.1075305

INDEX

2C-B, 139
5-MeO-DMT, 60

absorption, as a trait, 86–87
abuse. *See* exploitation; sexual boundaries
addiction, 89
adverse events, 78–100
See also challenges
aesthetics, 161–162
See also neuroaesthetics
afterglow, 95
agency, sense of, xxiii, 34, 86, 88, 230
Aixalà, M., 81, 259
alertness, relaxed, 72
altars, 163–164
American Association for Marriage and Family Therapy, 29
American Psychedelic Practitioners Association, 23, 134
American Psychological Association, 29, 31, 223
anarchic brain, 12–14, 15
ANS (autonomic nervous system), 229–232

Antelope Canyon, 159
arts and crafts, 270
See also drawing
art therapies, 153–154
attunement
  caregivers and, 232
  as a core competency, 111–112, 177–178
  Hakomi method and, 70
  soma and, 48
  therapeutic use of touch and, 211–213
  trauma and, 116–117
autobiographical memory, 246
autonomic nervous system (ANS), 229–232
avoidance, deprivation of touch and, 197
awake sacred spaces, 158–163
  See also space cleansing
awareness
  body, 130, 240
  inner state, 118–120
  mindful, 164–165
  pure, 114–115
  relational field, 112
  somatic, 62–63, 130
ayahuasca, 59, 91, 107, 151

bad trips. *See* adverse events
Bakalar, J., 96
basic goodness, 181
bipolar disorder, 123
blankets, 160, 162, 167, 205
    See also weighted blankets
blood pressure, elevated, 90
the body, 42–57
    See also *soma*
body awareness, 130, 240
    See also embodied presence; somatic awareness
body load, 49
body movement, 156–157, 239
    See also embodied movement; somatic movement
body narratives, 189–191, 217–218
    See also touch awareness
Bonny, H., 172
boosters, 142
borderline personality disorder (BPD), 124
bottom-up information processing, xxvi, 16–18, 61
    See also RElaxed Beliefs Under pSychedelics (REBUS); Somatic Experiencing (SE)
boundaries, 25–26, 28–30, 199, 284
    See also containing touch; informed consent
BPD (borderline personality disorder), 124
Bratman, G., 154
breathing, 63–64, 108–110
breathing patterns, 191
Brown, B., 274
bruxism, 91

Buddhist traditions, 158
building toward peak phase, 173
burnout, 228–229

canalization, 13
Carbonaro, T., 81
cardiovascular disease, 123
caregivers, 198, 232
Carhart-Harris, R., 12–13, 15
castle analogy, 133–134
cellphones, 188
Central Intelligence Agency (CIA), 19–20
challenges
    after journeys, 93–95, 133
    with integration, 254–256, 261
    during journeys, 80–82, 125, 234–240
    See also adverse events
client preparation
    about, 122–149
    exploring consent to touch in, 204–209
    pendulation from activation to resource, 236–237
    physiological adverse events and, 89–90
    trauma and, 233–234
clients. *See* journeyers
codes of ethics, 23
    See also ethics
collective trauma, 223
comedown, 173–174
community support, 256
compassion, 112
compassion heart, meeting your, 115–116
confidence, 108
confidentiality, 27, 40, 128

Conrad, E., 63
conscious breathing, 63–64
conscious orienting, 74–75
consent. *See* informed consent
"contact high," 21
containing touch, 203
Continuum, 63–64
contraindications, 11–12, 94, 122–123
coregulation, 64–65, 117, 187, 190
countertransference, 178–180
crazy, fear of going, 6, 93
creativity, 263, 269–270, 272
　See also journaling
curandera, 287

Damasio, A., 43
DEA (Drug Enforcement Administration), 283
de-canalization, 13
Descartes, R., xxv
developmental trauma, 223
Diagnostic and Statistical Manual of Mental Disorders (DSM-5), 96
directives. *See* language and directives, effects of
discharges, 132
dissociated sensory fragments, 245–246
dissociation, 124–125
DMT, 138–139
　See also ayahuasca
dosages, 88, 141–142
dosing sessions, logistics for, 143–144
downstream processing, 14–15
drala, 158–159
drawing, 263, 269
dreams, 181–182, 249–250
dreamwork, 268–270
drug choices, 136–140
　See also *specific drugs*

Drug Enforcement Administration (DEA), 283
drug interactions, 126–128
DSM-5 (Diagnostic and Statistical Manual of Mental Disorders), 96
Dune (Herbert), 132
dying, feeling of. *See* existential threats

earth-based cultures. *See* Indigenous traditions and wisdom
eating disorders, 124
ego dissolution, 155
ego inflation, 256
ego strength, 124, 182–183
Ekman, P., 266
embodied awakening, 217–218, 252–253
embodied cognition, 16
embodied movement, 267–268
　See also body movement; somatic movement
embodied presence, 111–112, 186, 191
embodiment, Western culture as dismissive of, 15–16
emergence, 171–172
emergency plans, 128
emotional integration, 265–267
emotional reciprocity, 232
　See also attunement
empathy and burnout, 228–229
emptying, 114
energy conservation, 229
energy release, intense, 217–218
epigenetics, 60–61
erotic countertransference, 179–180
erotic transference, 29–30
Ethical Principles/Code of Conduct (OHA), 23, 31

Ethical Principles of Psychologists and Code of Conduct (American Psychological Association), 29, 31
ethics, 19–41, 204, 285–286
Evans, J., 98
existential threats, 6, 92–93
expectations, 131–132, 215
  See also intentions, client's; intentions, therapist's
exploitation, 28–29, 284–285, 291
eyeshades, 143, 144

facial expressions and gestures, 190, 199–200
facilitating touch, 204
facilitators, xxii–xxiii, 136
  See also Somerville, P.; therapists
false memories, 236
family, friends, and community, 255–256
fatigue, 90
FDA (Food and Drug Administration), 19
fee structures, 128–129
felt sense, 47–49, 51, 113–114
  See also somatic markers
5-MeO-DMT, 60
fixity, 185–186
flashbacks, 95–97
  See also dissociated sensory fragments
Focusing (Gendlin), 48
Food and Drug Administration (FDA), 19
four Rs, 220–221
freewriting, 263
freeze response, 229–230
Freud, S., 181
friends, family, and community, 255–256

gastrointestinal issues, 90, 91, 123
  See also purging
Gendlin, E., 48

gestures and facial expressions, 190, 199–200
gnosis, 182
goodness, basic, 181
Grandfather Peyote, 290
gratitude, 278–279
Grinspoon, L., 96
Grof, C., 63
Grof, S., xxvi, 22, 35, 63, 92–93
grounded compassion, 112
grounding, 130, 173, 185
  See also guiding statements
ground rules, 134–135
guided inquiry, 64
guiding statements, 237

habit reinforcement, 272
Haines, S., 61
Hakomi method, xxvi, 17, 67–71, 76, 113
hallucinations, visual, 173, 182
hallucinogen-persisting perception disorder (HPPD), 96–97
Halpern, J., 97
hands-on touch, 203
harm reduction, xxii–xxiii, 9, 92
  See also ethics; therapeutic relationships
Harper, S., 63
headaches, 89–90
headphones, 143–144
heart rate, elevated, 90
heart rate variability (HRV), 187, 190
Hebb's Law, 13
helplessness, 230
Herbert, F., 132
hidden therapist, 163
higher power, 38
Hindu traditions, 218

history taking, 126–128, 205
Hofmann, A., 95
holding space for the inner healer, 112–113, 114–116
Holotropic Breathwork, 63
hózhó, 159
HPA (hypothalamic–pituitary–adrenal) axis, 231
HPPD (hallucinogen-persisting perception disorder), 96–97
HRV. *See* heart rate variability (HRV)
Huautla de Jiménez, Mexico, 288–289
humanistic psychology, 180
hypnotherapists, 20

ibogaine, 139
Indigenous traditions and wisdom
  avoiding exploitation of, 22
  divinity of psychedelics in, 289–291
  as earth-based cultures, 7–8
  integration practices and, 247
  reintegration of, 286–287
  rituals and setting in, 107, 152, 165–166
  through apprenticeships, 117–118
  See also Lakota traditions; Navajo traditions; shamanic traditions
inequality. *See* systemic inequality
informed consent
  about, 27
  adverse events, 89, 90, 98–100
  medical conditions, 123
  therapeutic use of touch, 204–209, 211–212
inner ethics, 24
inner healing intelligence, xxvi, 113, 184
inner state, awareness of, 118–120

intake checklists, 146–149
  See also screening and intake
integration, 75–77, 245–259, 265–267
  See also meaning making
integration sessions
  case studies, 210–211, 226–228, 274–277
  challenges during, 254–256, 261
  phases of, 262–263
  scheduling of, 143
  therapeutic tools for, 263–280
  therapeutic use of touch during, 218–219
  trauma and, 240–241
  value of, 250–252
intentions, client's, 131, 164, 264–265
intentions, therapist's, 117
intergenerational trauma, 34–35, 223–224
interoception, 46, 131, 183
interpersonal fields, 187–188
intervention, during adverse events, 82–86
intuition, 24, 192
investigatory reflex, 72
involuntary movements, 46
Iroquois Confederacy, 286

Johanson, G., 70
joining principle, 177–178
journaling, 263, 264, 271, 278, 279
journeyers
  caution against radical changes by, 256–257
  and challenges during integration phase, 254–256, 261
  and distress after a journey, 93–95
  ground rules for, 134–135
  insights from, xxvii, 14, 16, 181, 182

journeyers (*continued*)
  intentions and, 131, 164, 264–265
  and relief during integration, 251
  resistance and, 132
  spirituality and, 129, 248
  vulnerability of, 21, 274
  in Western culture, 8, 9
  See also therapeutic relationships
journeys
  attunement during, 177–178, 211–212
  case studies, 52–54, 210
  challenges after, 93–95, 133
  challenges during, 80–82, 125, 234–240
  countertransference during, 178–180
  ending, 194–195
  interoception during, 183
  interpersonal fields and, 187–188
  mindfulness during, 67–68, 176–177
  nonlinearity of, 174–176
  phases of, 172–174
  physical comfort during, 160–161, 162, 166–168, 188
  protection of, 188–189
  repetition and spacing of, 257–258
  as a series, 125–126
  therapeutic use of touch during, 173, 215–218
  trauma during, 234–240
  unconscious processing during, 180–183
judgment, 175–176, 177
Jung, C., 26, 268, 284

Kaelen, M., 172–174
kangaroo care, 198
karma, 175

ketamine, 51–54, 59, 140–141, 151
kundalini, 218
Kurtz, R., xxv, 67, 69

Lakota traditions, 114
language and directives, effects of, 193, 215, 230
Levine, P., xxv, xxvi, 71, 73, 74, 113, 184, 185, 193–194, 230
Life, 288
listening self-touch, 216–217
locus of control, 34
loneliness, 247
loving presence, 69
LSD
  about, 138
  dosages, 123
  effects of, 60
  ethics and, 20
  Grof on, 22
  Hofmann on, 95
  Sylvae's stepmother's story about, 78
LSD Psychotherapy (Grof), 35
Lüönd, A., 197

magic mushrooms, xiv, 137, 288
  See also psilocybin
Magsamen, S., 153
mandatory reporting, 27–28
Manson Family, 20
MAPS. *See* Multidisciplinary Association for Psychedelic Studies (MAPS)
marginalized groups, 34, 35
Maslow, A., 292
Maté, G., 224
materialism, spiritual, 291, 292
maturity, psychedelic-assisted therapy as initiation into, 301–302
Mazatec traditions, 152

MDMA
    about, 140, 141, 283
    contraindications for, 123
    effects of, 31, 59, 90, 91, 225
    Mithoefers on, 6–7
    PTSD and, 63
MDMA-assisted therapy (MDMA-AT), 19, 124, 142, 225, 283
meaning making, 232–233
    See also integration
medicine. *See* dosages; drug choices; *specific types*
Medusa and Perseus, 193–194
memories, false, 236
memories, repressed, 235–236
memory, autobiographical/narrative, 246
memory, procedural, 246
memory, state-dependent, 250
mental health disorders, 94–95, 123
mentors, 39–40
mescaline, 138
metta, 107
Metzner, R., 131
mind–body holism, 71
mindful awareness, 164–165
mindfulness, 67–68, 176–177, 240
Mischke-Reeds, M., xvii–xxi, xxv, 44–45, 47, 298–300
missing experience, 76
Mitchell, J., 225
Mithoefer, A., 6–7
Mithoefer, M., 6–7
modularity, 13–14
monsters, 193
movement, 46, 156–157, 160–161, 239, 267–268
    See also postures
multidimensional breathing, 108–110
multidimensional capacity, 110–111, 117–120
multidimensionality, 108–111
Multidisciplinary Association for Psychedelic Studies (MAPS), 6–7, 23, 63, 225
multiple relationships, 30–32
music, 143–145, 163, 173, 238, 270–271

narrative memory, 246
National Center for PTSD, 223
nature, connection to, 154–156, 159–160, 161
    See also Indigenous traditions and wisdom
nausea, 90, 123
    See also vomiting
Navajo traditions, 159
neuroaesthetics, 152–154
neuroception, 106–107
neuroplasticity, windows of, 12–13
nondirective approach, 17–18, 192
nonlinearity, of journeys, 174–176
non-maleficence, 92
nonviolence, 69
note taking, 189, 251
    See also body narratives

objective countertransference, 179
onset phase, 172–173
ontological shock, 254
openness, as a trait, 86–87
oppression. *See* systemic inequality
Oregon Health Authority (OHA), 23, 29, 31, 36
organicity, 70, 113
orienting, 74–75, 164, 215
oscillations. *See* pendulation
othering, 247
outer ethics, 24
oxytocin, 198

Pahnke, W., 172
parasympathetic nervous system, 229, 231
parts integration, 75–77
Pavlov, I., 72
payment. *See* fee structures
peak phase, 173
pendulation, 74, 183–186, 236–237
perceptual challenges. *See* hallucinogen-persisting perception disorder (HPPD)
Perls, F., 181
Perseus and Medusa, 193–194
Phelps, J., 111
physical space, 136, 150–168
physical transitions, 160–161
    See also body movement
physician consultation, 123–124, 127–128
physiological adverse events, 89–92
pillows, 160, 162, 167, 194, 205, 216
playlists, 144–145
Plotkin, B., 302
Pollan, M., 13
Porges, S., 106
positive psychology, 184, 185
posttraumatic growth, 224–225
posttraumatic stress disorder (PTSD)
    boosters in treatment of, 142
    connecting to nature and, 154
    demographics, 223
    dissociated sensory fragments and, 245–246
    ethics in treatment of, 19
    MAPS protocol and, 6, 225
    somatic awareness and, 63
postures, 190
power differentials, 32–33
pre-onset phase, 172

preparation phase, use of touch in, 213–215
preparation sessions, 129–135
    See also client preparation
prescribers, xxii
presence, 69, 111–112, 186, 191
procedural memory, 246
processing, 14–15, 66, 153, 180–183
    See also bottom-up information processing
Professional Practice Guidelines (APPA), 23
Project MKUltra program, 20
proprioception, 49
prosody, 190
pseudo-shamans, 284–285
psilocybin
    about, 137–138, 224
    dosages, 88
    effects of, xvii, xviii–xix, 31, 59
    history of, 287–289
    intervention due to adverse events from, 82–86
    repetition and spacing of journeys with, 257
    romantic and sexual boundaries, 29
psychedelic-assisted therapy
    about, 5–18
    benefits from, 10–11
    contraindications for, 11–12, 94, 122–123
    importance of legalization of, 283–284, 285
    as initiation into maturity, 301–302
    precautions for, xxi–xxii
    as uneconomical, 36
    See also client preparation; integration sessions; journeys; preparation sessions

psychedelic journeys, essentials of,
xxiii–xxiv
See also journeys
psychedelic materialism, 291
psychedelics
contraindications for, 174
defined, xxiv–xxv
divinity of, 289–291
drug interactions and, 126–128
mental health disorders and, 94–95,
123
soma and, 49–54
somatic psychotherapy and, 58–77
See also *specific medicines*
psychedelic therapists. *See* therapists
psychiatry, psychedelic-assisted therapy
versus, 9–10
psychological issues. *See* mental health
disorders
psychology, positive, 184, 185
psychopharmacology, 9
Psychopharmacology, 284
psychotic breaks, 94
psychotropic cures, 9
pure awareness, 114–115
purging, 59, 60, 91, 124

reassurance, 76, 173, 188, 189
reassuring touch, 202–203
reentry phase, 173–174
reflection, 271
See also integration sessions;
journaling
regression, 21
relational field, awareness of the, 112,
177
relationships, 29–32
See also therapeutic relationships
relaxed alertness, 72

RElaxed Beliefs Under pSychedelics
(REBUS), 15
renegotiation, 245
repressed memories, 235–236
resilience
challenging experiences and, 81–82
embodiment practices and, 61–62
gratitude and, 278–279
preparation phase and assessment of,
124
somatic markers and, 45
therapist's role in, 38
touch and, 197
trusting the soma and, 54–55
resistance, 132
resources, 64, 185, 236–237, 240–241
return phase, 174
Richards, W., 137
Rinpoche, C., 181, 291
risks and complications, 132–135
See also contraindications; drug
interactions
rituals, 107, 152, 165–166, 172, 272
ritual spaces, 163–165
Rogers, C., 180
romantic relationships, 29–30

Sabina, M., 287–289
sacred spaces, 152, 163, 164, 165–166
See also awake sacred spaces
SAEs (serious adverse events), 79
safety
body load and, 49–50
in dealing with overwhelm, 193–194
at end of journey, 195
investigatory reflex and, 72
marginalization and, 34
physical space and, 157–158, 162
sequencing and, 65–66

safety (continued)
  somatic markers and, 56
  tracking and, 105–106
  See also neuroception; somatic set and setting
schizophrenia, 94, 123
screening and intake, 122–129
  See also intake checklists
SE. See Somatic Experiencing (SE)
The Secret Chief Revealed (Zeff), 133
self, sense of, 197
  See also presence
self-acceptance, 252–253, 255
self-efficacy, 34
self-touch, 213–214, 216–217
Selver, C., 62
sensation seeking, 125
sensory awareness, 62
sensory fragments, dissociated, 245–246
sequencing, 65–66
serious adverse events (SAEs), 79
serotonin syndrome, 127
set and setting, 85–86, 104–107, 151
  See also physical space
sexual boundaries, 28–29, 284
shadow, 26, 248, 255
shamanic traditions, 39, 91, 93, 165
shamans, xxii, 290–291
  See also pseudo-shamans
Shambhala approach, 158
shame, 26, 255, 274–278
  See also shadow
Shepard, P., 248, 302
shock trauma, 223
Shulgin, A., 139, 140
side effects. See adverse events
sites of shaping and change, 61
sitters, xxii

slow processing, 66
social engagement system, 231–232
soma, 42–43, 48–55, 58–59
somatic awareness, 62–63, 130
Somatic Experiencing (SE), xxvi, 17, 71–75, 84–86
somatic intelligence, 61–62
somatic markers, 43–46, 55–56, 57
somatic movement, 160–161
  See also body movement; embodied movement
somatic opening, 118–120
somatic psychology, 43
somatic psychotherapy, psychedelics and, 58–77
somatic resources, 64
somatic set and setting, 104–107
somatic therapists, 43, 62, 303
  See also therapists
somatic tracking, 66–67, 173
somatosensory distortions, 49, 173, 174
  See also dissociated sensory fragments
Somerville, P., 82–85
soundproofing, 162–163
space. See physical space
space cleansing, 165–166
speech qualities, 190–191
spiritual bypassing, 261
spirituality, 129, 248
spiritual materialism, 291, 292
Spitz, R., 197
SSRIs, 127
Starhawk, 33
state-dependent memory, 250
stillness, 272–274
stress reduction
  conscious breathing and, 63

neuroception and, 106
social engagement system and, 231
through neuroaesthetics and nature, 153–156
touch and, 197, 198
stress response, 106, 157, 198
subjective countertransference, 179
subpersonalities, 75
suicidal ideation, 97–98, 124
supervision, 39–40
support, community, 256, 257
surrendering, 230
Sweeney, M., 224
Sylvae, J., xiii–xvii, xxv, 31, 78, 293–298
sympathetic nervous system, 229, 231
systemic inequality, 32–36

tachycardia, 90
Taoism, 114–115
Taylor, K., 24
technology, 188
texts, 188
therapeutic relationships
    components of, 175–180, 181, 184, 185–188
    nondirective approach, 17–18, 192
    power differentials in, 32–33
    precautions for, 21–22
    preconditions for, 21
    See also harm reduction
therapeutic use of touch
    about, 135–136
    attunement and, 211–213
    case study, 210–211
    consent in use of, 204–209, 211–212
    ethics and, 23, 204, 208–209
    four Rs, 220–221
    as grounding, 173

guidelines for, 201–202
during integration sessions, 218–219
during journeys, 173, 215–218
in preparation phase, 213–215
types of, 202–204
See also touch awareness
therapist preparation, 103–121
See also therapist training
therapists
    and confidentiality as a practitioner, 27, 40, 128
    consideration of own ethics and motives by, 24–25
    core competencies of, 111–114, 177–178
    effects of language and directives used by, 193, 215, 230
    empathy and burnout in, 228–229
    experiential ethics for, 37–38
    exploitation by, 285–286
    journey experience of, 251–252
    as multidimensional, 108–111
    oversight for, 39–40
    responses to suffering by, 87
    trauma within the journey and strategies for, 239–240
    See also facilitators; therapeutic relationships
therapist training, 7, 9, 39–40
Tibetan Buddhist traditions, 158
titration, 73
TOMI (Touch Outcomes Measurement Inventory), 219
tonglen, 107
touch, 196–199
    See also self-touch; therapeutic use of touch
touch awareness, 199–201

tracking
  consent and, 212
  in the journey phase, 189–191, 217
  mindfulness and, 176
  safety and, 105–106
  somatic, 66–67
  See also somatic markers; somatic tracking
traits, 86–87
transference, 29–30, 134–135
transitions, physical, 160–161
  See also body movement
trauma
  ANS and, 229–232
  becoming informed about, 116–117
  case study, 226–228
  continuum of, 223–224
  dissociated sensory fragments in, 245–246
  epigenetics and, 60–61
  integration phase and, 240–241
  intergenerational, 34–35, 223–224
  journey phase and occurrence of, 234–240
  Levine's approach to healing, 193–194
  meaning making and, 232–233
  preparation phase and, 233–234
  Somatic Experiencing (SE) and, 71–74
  as transformative, 224–225
  See also posttraumatic stress disorder (PTSD)
trauma vortex, 74
treatment rooms, 136
  See also physical space
tripsitters, xxii

Tronick, E., 232
true self, 249
trust building. See somatic set and setting
trusting the process, 54–55
Tsé Bíghanílíní, 159
2C-B, 139

unconditional positive regard, 180
unconscious processing, 180–183
unity, 70

via regia, 181–182
visual hallucinations, 173, 182
visual processing, 153
voice quality, 190
vomiting, 91, 123
vulnerability
  power differentials and, 32
  psychedelics and, 12, 21, 173, 255
  therapeutic use of touch and, 203
  touch awareness and, 199
  trauma and, 230
vulnerability hangover, 274

Waking the Tiger (Levine), 193
walking yourself home, 300–301
Wasson, R., 288–289
weighted blankets, 162, 194, 216
WEIRD countries, 8
Welwood, J., 261
Western culture
  as dismissive of embodiment, 15–16
  issues causing fragmentation within, 247–248
  and lack of humility for primary cultures, 286–289
  lack of preparation for psychedelic-assisted therapy in, 8, 9

power differentials in, 32–33
psychedelic renaissance in, 5–7, 22
somatic markers and, 44
systemic inequality and, 32–36
training style in, 118
windows of neuroplasticity, 12–13

Winnicott, D., 249
writing, 269–270
 See also freewriting; journaling
wu wei, 114–115

Zeff, L., 133–134

ABOUT THE AUTHORS

Manuela Mischke-Reeds, MFT, is a somatic trauma psychotherapist, author, and internationally respected teacher of somatic psychology and Continuum. She is the founder of Embodywise and the Hakomi Institute of California, as well as the creator of Innate Somatic Intelligence Trauma Therapy (ISITTA), an integrative, somatic approach to trauma healing. With over 25 years of clinical experience, Manuela has worked with a wide range of trauma survivors, including refugees, first responders, and survivors of political violence. As core faculty in the Hakomi Method, she brings a compassionate, embodied lens to healing, blending movement, mindfulness, and nervous system science. Manuela teaches internationally on trauma-informed care, somatic psychedelic therapy, and movement-based healing. Her books include *Trauma-Sensitive Movement, Somatic Psychotherapy Toolbox,* and *8 Keys to Practicing Mindfulness.* Through her teaching and writing, she invites practitioners and clients alike into deeper safety, presence, and transformation. Learn more at embodywise.com and manuelamischkereeds.com.

Joshua Sylvae, PhD, is a licensed marriage and family therapist from Oregon. His work as a helper focuses on somatic practice, nature-based healing, trauma recovery, and expanded states of consciousness. He teaches the Somatic Experiencing Professional Training around the world, facilitates master classes for Peter Levine's Ergos Institute of Somatic Education, and leads private workshops. He is certified in psychedelic-assisted therapy and has trained in MDMA-assisted therapy for PTSD. He founded the (r)evolve Foundation, a 501(c)(3) nonprofit dedicated to educating the public about human origins and stimulating dialogue about the mismatch between our biology and our civilized environments. He is a musician, a lover of wilderness, and is dedicated to his relationships with his family and community. Currently, Joshua is dreaming about a podcast and—in any spare moments he can carve out—writing on multiple topics.